# Examination of the Eye
# Made Easy

# Examination of the Eye Made Easy

John C. Barber, MD, FAAO

**To order additional copies of this book, contact:**
Xlibris
844-714-8691
www.Xlibris.com
Orders@Xlibris.com
852046

# CONTENTS

# About the Author

Dr. John C. Barber studied engineering and premedical studies at Purdue University before graduating from Washington University Medical School in St. Louis. After a rotating internship and two years in the Food and Drug Administration, he did a combined clinical and research NIH-sponsored residency in Ophthalmology at the Medical College of Virginia. He then specialized in the front half of the eye by doing a fellowship with Dr. Claes H. Dohlman at Massachusetts Eye and Ear Infirmary (Harvard Medical School) in Boston, where he was an instructor in ophthalmology.

Dr. Barber's next academic position was at the University of Texas Medical Branch in Galveston where he taught medical students and ophthalmology residents. He was department chairman there for nine years, running a major ophthalmology residency program, doing research, and seeing private patients. He then moved to Pittsburgh to become department chairman and director of the ophthalmology residency program at St. Francis Medical Center. He also served as director of medical education for seven residency programs at that institution. He was CEO of St. Francis Eye associates, Inc., the corporation that supported the Ophthalmology Residency.

Throughout his career, Dr. Barber was an active participant in teaching physical diagnosis of the eye to medical students and resident physicians.

During thirty years of academic medicine as a hands-on residency program director and department chairman, he was largely responsible for training more than ninety ophthalmologists.

Throughout his medical career he conducted a private referral practice specializing in the front half of the eye, especially corneal transplants.

While in Texas, he conducted several research projects including the development a retainable corneal prosthesis (artificial cornea).

# Examination of the Eye and Adnexa

## Introduction

It is incumbent on every physician to be able to examine the eye and its adnexa. The eye may contain signs of many diseases that involve the entire body and the evidence needed to confirm the diagnosis that was suspected from the medical history and other parts of the physical examination of the body.

Because the eye contains nerves, vessels, muscles, pigmented tissues, and connective tissues derived from each of three embryonic layers, diseases that affect any of these tissues may cause changes in the eye. Both sensory and motor nerves have extensive roles in the movement and function of the eye.

The eye is the only place in the body where blood vessels can be seen and evaluated.

Patients with diabetes mellitus often have changes in the vessels of the retina as well as hemorrhages, exudates and infarcts within the retina. Diabetes is also the cause of palsies of the eye muscles and decrease in the visual acuity because of cataracts and retinal edema.

Hypertensive patients will have changes in the diameter of retinal arteries and pinching of the veins where they share a common muscular coat with arteries at vessel crossings. Hemorrhages within the retina from arterial hypertension have a characteristic shape and distribution.

Atherosclerosis of the arteries causes another characteristic change in the crossings of the blood vessels of the retina. Atherosclerosis causes the vessel walls to become opaque and obscure the blood in veins behind the arteries at artery-vein crossings resulting in a gap in the view of the venous blood that is wider that the bloodstream within the artery. The findings of hypertension and atherosclerosis may both be present simultaneously.

Forward protrusion of one or both eyes may be caused by malignant or benign tumors, bone changes, vascular anomalies, or thyroid disease prompting further examination and testing. Thyroid disease may affect any or all of the extraocular muscles.

Many other systemic diseases (i.e., lupus erythematosus, sarcoidosis, tuberculosis, fat emboli, and septicemia) have specific findings within the eye, eyelids, and orbit that can contribute to the correct diagnosis. Myasthenia gravis often presents with ptosis (drooping) of one eyelid or intermittent double vision related to weakness of extra-ocular muscles, but it must not be confused with partial paralysis of the third cranial nerve from diabetes or hypertension.

The findings within the eye may suggest a diagnosis of AIDS or ARCS that may lead to partial or total blindness if not discovered and treated before they become advanced.

The physician who does not examine the eye, both inside and out, does his patient and himself a major disservice.

# The Basic External Eye Exam

## Visual Acuity

The initial activity in determining the function of the eye is the determination of visual acuity. This is classically determined by comparing the accuracy of central vision with the norm. This part of the exam is often relegated to a nurse or technician who must be trained to perform the test correctly to obtain reliable results.

The patient is asked to read letters or to name objects depicted on a chart, either on the wall or in the hands of the examiner or the patient. The light receptive cone cells (think of them as pixels) are tightly packed in the macula, so the distance between a cone that is being stimulated by light and one that is not is very small, making edges distinct for small letters or objects. When some cones are not functioning correctly, the distance between working cones is greater, so edges are blurred and images must be larger for recognition. Similarly, when the image is not in focus, the edges are indistinct and contrasts are blurred.

The letters on the 20/20 line of the chart are the size that a normal person, with normally-spaced functioning cones, can distinguish at a distance of twenty feet from the eye. The 20/40 letters are twice as large so they make the same size image on the retina when viewed at forty feet from the eye as the 20/20 letters make at twenty feet. The 20/200 letters are ten times larger than the 20/20 letters. Some charts have a 20/400 letter at the top which is twice as large as the 20/200 letter. Europeans and some Americans use six meters rather than twenty feet so 6/6 is equal to 20/20 and 6/60 is equal to 20/200.

The visual acuity near card uses the same geometry to create numbers or letters that have the same retinal image size as the twenty-foot chart when the card is held at fourteen (14) inches from the eye.

Since some people have sharper acuity than 20/20, these charts have lines of letters that are smaller than the 20/20 letters. These are usually 20/15 and 20/10 lines.

> Although some patients can read these smaller lines flawlessly, I reported vision of 20/10 on a navy pilot's visual exam and had it returned by the navy with a letter stating that 20/20 vision was normal and therefore better vision was impossible, so the report must be corrected to 20/20. Bureaucracy over science!
>
> Normal vision is considered to be 20/20 unless documented to be otherwise. A chemical burn patient who read the 20/20 line after recovering from the injury claimed that he had had better vision before his accident and wanted compensation for his loss. No one had ever documented his better vision, i.e. 20/15 or 20/10. Since 20/20 is considered normal, he was not allowed any compensation.

The Importance of Visual Acuity Testing

The measure of visual acuity gives an approximation of the limitations of activity level caused by visual impairment. Normal vision is 20/20, but not all eyes are capable of this visual level because of various diseases or malformations. Most people are able to function normally with vision equal to, or better than, 20/40. Most states require vision of 20/40 or better to be allowed to drive a car. Some states allow day-time, non-highway driving with vision equal or better than 20/70. This applies to the best vision obtainable with glasses or contact lenses in either eye called best corrected vision. If visual correction (glasses or contact lenses) is necessary to obtain this level of vision, the license is marked with a code indicating that correction must be worn while driving.

Many states have laws requiring physicians to report patients who have vision less than 20/40 to the department of motor vehicles with fines to the physician for not reporting, if the patient is involved in a traffic accident. Some states go so far as to declare the physician financially responsible for the accident.

Airline pilots must have vision correctable to 20/20 in both eyes with both eyes working together to provide adequate depth perception. Accountants may begin making mistakes in reading numbers before their vision decreases to the 20/40 level, while some people with vision levels as low as 20/200 can function adequately, if they are familiar with the tasks they perform during normal daily living, as long as it does not include driving, flying, or significant amounts of reading. Low vision aids that magnify print can make limited amounts of reading possible for the partially sighted.

Fortunately, the leading cause of vision that is worse than 20/20 is the eye being out of focus. This can be corrected by glasses. Best corrected vision that is less than 20/20 may indicate eye disease. One of the most common causes of eye disease in older adults is cataract—clouding of the lens in the eye.

Surgical decisions are often made on the basis of visual acuity. Insurance companies may deny payment for cataract surgery that does not meet their standards of need (decreased visual acuity). Generally, surgery should usually be delayed or denied if the risks of a bad result are considered more than the expected visual improvement can justify.

Several years ago, some insurance companies in New Jersey would not pay for cataract removal unless the best corrected vision with glasses, or contact lenses, was 20/70 or worse before surgery. At the same time, the Department of Motor Vehicles required vision of 20/40 to maintain a driver's license. What were people to do who were between 20/40 and 20/70 in the maturation of their cataracts? People did not want to wait the months to years while the cataract slowly matured. The insurance companies soon changed their policies to vision of 20/40 or worse.

Testing Visual Acuity

To determine visual acuity, each eye is examined separately. The other eye is occluded with an opaque card or occluder. The patient may hold a hand over the eye not being tested, but the examiner must be sure that the palm of the hand is used, not the fingers. Small cracks or peepholes between the fingers may act as a pin hole, or stenopeic slit, that actually improves the vision of the eye being occluded rather than blocking vision.

The patient reads the chart, or the near card, from top to bottom until they cannot read the letters. Some near cards contain text rather than letters or numbers. This gives a better evaluation of reading impairment. Vision for that eye is recorded as the label on the chart for that line (i.e., 20/30). In the record, the vision recorded may state the number of letters read correctly on the last line or the number missed, whichever is least. g., 20/40 + 2 (on the 20/30 line) or 20/40 – 1 (1 missed on the 20/40 line.)

Vision is usually recorded with a large letter *V* followed by the acuity for each eye. By convention, the vision for the right eye is recorded above the vision for the left eye.

$$V \quad \begin{array}{l} 20/30 + 2 \text{ OD } (ocular\ dextra) \\ 20/20 - 1 \text{ OS } (ocular\ sinistra) \end{array}$$

This part of the exam may be shortened, if there is no reason to suspect poor vision, by directing the patient to start reading the chart at the 20/40 line. If this is difficult, the examiner may always instruct the patient to go to a higher line.

Checking the vision with both eyes open simultaneously is not done because it only measures the best acuity in either eye. It could be slightly better than either eye due to fusion of the two images by the brain, but does not indicate the vision in each eye. One eye could have poorer acuity.

Special Cases

A patient with the unusual condition called dissociated vertical deviation (DVD) can be difficult to measure visual acuity in each eye. In this condition, when one eye is covered, both eyes move upward behind the upper eyelids and do not look at the acuity chart. This upward movement is not under the control of the patient. If only the central vision is blocked in one eye, without blocking the peripheral vision, the eyes will stay directed toward the acuity chart, providing that both eyes have relatively good vision. Something narrow like a pencil, or split tongue blade, can be held in front of the pupil of one eye to block that eye from reading the chart while peripheral vision in that eye keeps the eyes from moving vertically.

Patients with high astigmatism may tilt their head to one side to sharpen their vision. When the axis of the astigmatism is aligned with the vertical (90°) or horizontal (180°) axis, the distortion becomes symmetrical and chart is easier to read. In cases with head tilt, it is best to obtain the vision with the head held straight and again in the patients preferred position. Correction of the astigmatism with glasses or contact lenses may eliminate the head tilt.

Visual acuity charts are also made with numbers for use with the alphabetically illiterate. Patients, including small children, can be taught the tumbling E game. They are taught to point in the direction of the open end of the E on the E chart as the examiner uses a blank card with a hole in it to expose one E at a time on the chart or points to the letter. Square cardboard boxes with different sized letter E on each side can be held by the examiner and turned in different directions to better hold the child's attention.

Another chart that is used for children and illiterate adults uses line drawings of familiar objects like a birthday cake or a boat. This drawing uses varying boldness of lines and changes in object size to measure the visual acuity.

When testing with a wall chart and exposing one letter at a time, it is possible for people with amblyopia (lazy eye) to read more letters when viewing single letters than when reading from a whole line of letters. Patients with amblyopia experience the phenomenon of "crowding" with multiple letters, which makes the letters harder to see than when they are viewed singly.

Driver's license offices and screening clinics use visual acuity equipment, such as a Titmus screener, to simulate distance vision in small spaces. These instruments use lenses to block focusing (accommodation) to simulate distance vision. Young patients (less than forty years old) may focus anyway because they are conscious that the letters they are looking at are inside the small instrument. This focusing, when added to the lenses in the device, causes blurring of the letters, giving falsely poor vision results. These devices work well on patients older than forty-five or fifty years old.

Failing the vision test for a driver's license usually results in being sent with a form to an eye doctor for formal verification of the patient's vision and correction with glasses or contact lenses, if helpful, to maximize visual acuity.

For driving, most states also require a horizontal visual field range of 100° for a one centimeter object while both eyes open. This requirement may be satisfied with only one eye if the field is normal in that eye (i.e., 20° nasal plus 80° temporal). A one-eyed person may obtain a driver's license in most states if the eye is normal without glasses or is correctable with glasses to 20/40 or better. Depth perception is not required in most states for a driver's license.

If the patient has myopia (nearsightedness), hyperopia (farsightedness), or astigmatism (distorted vision) and does not have optical correction with spectacles or contact lenses to correct the condition, the possible corrected vision that could be obtained with optical correction may be approximated by having the patient look through a pinhole. This can be a hole made by a safety pin or paper clip in a card or professionally with the multiple holes in a pinhole occluder. The pinhole works on the principle of the pinhole camera. It narrows the aperture for light so that focusing of multiple rays is not needed to form a clear image on the retina. Visual acuity obtained in this manner is denoted by the letters *P* and *H* next to the recorded vision. Patients may have 20/20 PH vision, even though they see poorly without glasses. This usually means that the only problem with vision is the need for optical correction with glasses or contact lenses.

A patient who is over the age of forty-five may need a pinhole or reading glasses to read the near visual acuity card. These older patients should wear their glasses with near correction, if they have them available, when being checked for visual acuity.

Interesting Fact

Automated visual acuity devices can be used to check the patient's vision without them reading a chart. NASA developed a system using projected moving lines to produce optokinetic nystagmus. The eye movements were detected with electrodes to the right and left of the eye to measure the movement of the positive charge of the front of the eyeball.

The width of the lines is decreased until the lines become too thin for the subject to see, so the nystagmus stops. The line width at which optokinetic nystagmus ceased has been correlated with visual acuity using normal subjects. With this device, the visual acuity of the astronaut could be measured by having them press their face into the device to watch the lines until they disappeared. Each eye is tested separately. This system has not been incorporated into ophthalmology practices.

An ophthalmologist, using a spot or streak retinascope, can determine need for and the correct power for optical correction on an illiterate person or infant. The light from the retinascope is shown into the eye through the lenses held before the eye. Movement of the light reflection in the pupil tells the ophthalmologist to increase or decrease the power of the lens until the movement is neutralized by the correct lens. By moving the spot or streak in various directions, the axis and amount of astigmatism can be measured for a total optical correction.

There are many excellent books on the theory and practice of refraction of the eye for visual correction, so refraction is not covered in this book.

# The Screening Examination

The typical examination of the eyes begins during the medical history interview of the patient. It is important to make eye contact with the patient to establish rapport with the patient. Whether the eyes are open equally and looking at the same object should be immediately apparent.

The color of the irises should be the same in both eyes. Differences in the pupil size between the eyes may, or may not, be apparent by casual viewing. Swelling, bruising, hemorrhages, abrasions, and lacerations as well as abnormal pigmentation may be observed during the taking of the history.

(History is the backbone of the evaluation of the patient. For the significance of signs and symptoms of eye disease see *Hey Doc! What's Wrong With My Eye: A General Guide to Eye Systems* by John C Barber, MD. 2017, Xlibris, Bloomington, Indiana.)

## Penlight Examination

The best way to start the examination of the eye is with the patient seated on the examination table or exam chair with the examiner seated or standing in front of the patient with a penlight in one hand.

## Ocular Alignment

The patient is asked to look at the light while it is held directly in front of the patient's face about two to three feet away. The examiner looks down the beam of light at the eyes to see if they are both looking at the light. If both eyes are looking at the light, there will be a small spot of light reflection on the cornea caused by the penlight. This spot should be just nasal to the center of the pupil and symmetrically located in both eyes. Asymmetry of the location of this spot with respect to the pupil indicates that one eye is not looking at the light. Depending on the cause and duration of the asymmetry, the patient may experience double vision. Further evaluation will be covered later.

Eye Movement

The eyes are observed for spontaneous movement. Nystagmus (rhythmical oscillation of the eyeballs) can be induced or can occur spontaneously. Nystagmus may occur normally in the extremes of horizontal gaze.

> This is accentuated with toxicity from drugs or alcohol, so following an object to the extreme left or right with the face straight ahead is used by police as part of the roadside sobriety test.

Nystagmus, that is involuntary, rhythmically repeated oscillations of one or both eyes may be congenital or acquired. In congenital "jerk" nystagmus, there is a fast component in one direction with a slow recovery movement in the opposite direction. The amount of the movement varies with the position of the eyes (right, left, or somewhere in between) with one position of gaze where it is least. This point is called the null point.

Children who have lost all vision or are significantly impaired before the age of two develop a searching nystagmus in which the eye wanders back and forth randomly.

Covering one eye may induce nystagmus in both eyes, which stops when the cover is removed. This is called latent nystagmus.

There are many forms of nystagmus related to neurologic diseases, including downbeat, upbeat, seesaw, alternating, gaze-evoked, and vestibular. These forms are rare and the causes are beyond the scope of this book. They can be diagnosed by a neurologist or neuro-ophthalmologist.

Optokinetic nystagmus (OKN) is normal and can be induced by repetitive moving objects, such as telephone poles seen from a moving car or by a train going past. This is replicated clinically by lines, figures, or pictures on a rotating drum or contrasting lines or squares on a strip of cloth or paper (e.g., a measuring tape), which is drawn past the eyes. The rotating drum is used as a test for malingering. OKN can be suppressed by staring past the moving objects, so the examiner must watch the eyes of the patient to be sure that they are looking at the moving targets.

> I have heard that the army used pictures of scantily
> clad women on the rotating drum to assure focusing
> on the rotating images when testing for malingering
> blindness to avoid military service.

Nystagmus can also be induced by stimulation of the normal middle ear by rotating the patient in a rotating chair or by stimulation with hot or cold water irrigated into the ear canal. The direction of the fast component of the nystagmus depends on the temperature of the irrigated water--*cold* water induces nystagmus with a fast component toward the *opposite* side; *warm* water causes the fast component toward the *same* side as the stimulated ear. Memory aid: COWS.

After examining the eye at rest, the patient is asked to keep watching the light as the light is brought toward the patient's nose. The eyes should turn inward to follow the light and the point of light reflection should stay within the pupil. In a few patients, this may elicit nystagmus as the light approaches the nose, which is considered a normal variant. At some point, the eyes may refuse to converge further, at which point one eye, or both, will return to straight ahead position. If this occurs more than one foot from the eye, the patient may have ocular convergence insufficiency.

In patients near or over the age of forty, the image may blur from age-induced lack of accommodation (presbyopia), making it more difficult for the patient to hold convergence. Patients who have had multiple concussions and divers with repeated episodes of "the Bends" lose the ability to converge. The pupil should constrict as the penlight, or other object used as the point of gaze, becomes close to the patient, causing the patient to accommodate (focus up close).

The light is held in front of the patient again and the patient is asked to follow the light. The examiner moves the light from right to left and back taking the gaze to extreme right and left. The examiner watches the eyes to see if they follow the light. Failure of one eye to follow the light may indicate a weakness of an ocular muscle, damage to the nerve controlling that muscle, or some physical restraint of the eyeball.

Sixth nerve palsy causes inability to abduct the eye (move away from midline toward the temporal side). Thyroid disease may affect any ocular muscle, decreasing its ability to stretch. This may result in strange eye movements.

Extraocular Muscles

The light is then moved into the cardinal positions of gaze (right, left, straight up, straight down, up and right, down and right, up and left and down and left), watching to see if the eyes always follow the light.

During this maneuver, the eyelids move up and down with the eyeball, allowing the eyelids to almost close when the eyes are in down gaze. To see the eyes move, it may be necessary to hold the eyelids up. This can be accomplished by placing the heel of the hand that is not holding the light upon the forehead of the patient and elevating the eyelids with the thumb and index fingers. The skin of the eyelids is lifted and held gently against the upper orbital rim, holding the eyes open.

Right and left gaze check the horizontal rectus muscles (medial and lateral rectus). Up and down gaze check the superior and inferior rectus muscles and the superior and inferior oblique muscles. Up and out and down and out gaze evaluate the function of the oblique muscles.

Inability to abduct (move away from the nose) either eye would indicate a problem with the abducens nerve [CN VI] or the lateral rectus muscle. Damage to the sixth cranial nerve is the most common of the ocular nerve palsies. It is the longest of the nerves controlling eye movements and has the most causes of injury, including trauma, diabetes, hypertension, increased intracranial pressure, brain tumors, metastases, vascular disease, and meningitis.

Damage to the trochlear nerve [CN IV] affects only the superior oblique muscle which pulls the axis of the eye down and out. Paralysis of this muscle allows the inferior oblique muscle to move the eye up and out, but the eye will not move down and out. The most common cause of fourth nerve palsy is trauma, especially frontal blows to the head (e.g., running into a wall or door or hitting the dashboard of a car). Other causes are vascular, including hypertension and diabetes.

The oculomotor nerve [CN III] serves the remaining rectus muscles (superior, inferior, and medial), the inferior oblique muscle, and the levator muscle to the upper eyelid that opens the eye. It also causes constriction of the pupil. Damage to the third nerve leaves the eyelid with ptosis or completely closed. When the eyelid is opened by the examiner, the eye looks down and out. The pupil may be dilated or normal. A third nerve palsy with a reactive pupil is more common when the cause is diabetes or hypertension, whereas a third nerve palsy with a nonreactive (dilated) pupil is indicative of pressure on the nerve from a tumor or aneurysm of the circle of Willis. The other common cause is trauma.

Having the patient watch the light as it moves up and down allows the examiner to observe whether the eyelid moves with the eyeball. It should. Conditions like myasthenia gravis may cause the eyelid to lag behind the eye. With prolonged up gaze, the eyelid that originally appeared normal may droop and cover the pupil. In hyperthyroid disease, the eyelid may overshoot and retract, showing white sclera between the eyelid and the cornea. When the light is brought down, the lid may lag behind and lower in a jerky fashion.

Thyroid eye disease may affect the extraocular muscles either singly, or in combinations, giving movements that do not fit a neurological pattern. Regeneration of a damaged CN III may cause abnormal eye and lid movements.

Congenital strabismus (abnormal ocular alignment and movements) may give patterns other than pure nerve damage. These will be discussed under cover testing.

The Iris and Pupil

With penlight still in hand, the patient is asked to look straight ahead. The light is shown into the pupil of one eye along, or near to, the axis of the eye, directed to shine on the central retina while the pupil is watched for movement. The light is withdrawn by moving it to the side before presenting it again. (Shine the light on the ear.) The pupil should constrict when light is shown into the eye and dilate when the light is removed. This pupil movement is called the direct pupillary light response.

This light movement is repeated while the examiner watches the pupil of the other eye. The pupil not being illuminated should constrict along with the pupil into which the light is shown and then dilate again when the light is withdrawn. This is called the indirect or consensual pupillary light response.

The direct pupillary response depends on the optic nerve and the third cranial nerve on the ipsilateral side. The consensual response depends of the optic nerve from the stimulated eye and the third cranial nerve on the contralateral side. Testing both sides allows the examiner to determine in which nerve and on which side the defect lies.

If the eye is completely blind, but the light response is present, the blindness is caused by a problem posterior to the lateral geniculate bodies at the base of the brain, such as cortical blindness. Cortical blindness can be caused by trauma to the back of the head or hypotension during surgery in which the patient is positioned face downward.

Disease of the optic nerve may cause a decrease in the degree and briskness of pupillary constriction. To detect this small difference, the penlight is moved repeatedly back and forth from right to left eye while watching the pupils. The pupil on the damaged side will appear to dilate slightly when the light is shown in that pupil and constrict when the other eye is illuminated. This is called the swinging flashlight test, and the dilation of the effected pupil is called the afferent nerve defect. (CN II is the afferent nerve and CN III is the efferent nerve in this reflex.)

Next, without the light shining directly into the eye, the patient is asked to look at a distant object more than five feet away and then at an object about one foot in front of the eye, such as a near card, and then back to distance while the pupil is observed. The pupil should constrict as gaze shifts from far to near and dilate as gaze shifts from near to distance. An object that requires focusing, like a near card and a wall vision chart, must be used. The eye does not have to focus on a light at near or far, so the constriction may not occur. The patient must intentionally look at both the far object and the near object to cause the eye to focus (accommodate).

As the eye accommodates to focus at different distances, the size of the pupil changes. This is part of the synkinetic near response (accommodation, convergence of the eyes, and constriction of the pupil). This pupil reaction is called the accommodative pupillary response. A small pupil has greater depth of field or range of objects in focus. Patients with neurosyphilis lose the ability to constrict the pupil to light, but retain the ability to constrict with accommodation. The classic memory tool is "The syphilitic pupil is like a prostitute; it accommodates, but does not react."

In patients with very dark irises, it may be difficult to see the pupil. In these cases, the iris may be illuminated from the side, obliquely, to be able to see the pupil movement as the eye accommodates.

Anterior Chamber Depth

While the penlight is still in hand, the depth of the anterior chamber of the eye (space between the cornea and the iris) can be determined by shining the light toward the eye, from the side of the eye, in the plane of the iris, while observing the light pattern on the surface of the iris. The light is slowly brought forward toward the examiner while still shining on the iris (rotating around the eye). If the iris is flat as it normally is, the whole surface, from temporal to nasal, will be lighted as soon as the penlight is anterior to the plane of the iris (sunrise on the flat prairie). If the iris is bowed forward, the light will only shine on the temporal side of the iris until the light is brought forward enough to shine over the anterior dome of the iris to illuminate the nasal side (sunrise in the mountains).

The iris is usually flat and the cornea is dome shaped, so iris that is bowed forward would indicate a shallow anterior chamber that may be susceptible to glaucoma attacks. This pupil should not be dilated with mydriatic eye drops until it has been examined by an ophthalmologist to determine if the angle is open sufficiently, all of the way to the trabecular meshwork, and is, therefore, not susceptible to closure by dilation that would precipitate a glaucoma attack.

The External Eyeball

The penlight is useful in examination of the external eye, especially in dimly lighted examination rooms and hospital rooms. Spreading the eyelids with the thumb and forefinger of one hand and illuminating the eye with the penlight in the other hand allows a good examination of the conjunctiva and the eyeball. The thumb is placed on the cheek below the eye and pulled down with light pressure on the cheek bone. The index finger is used to push the upper eyelid skin up over the brow to lift the lid margin. The lid is held in position with gentle pressure against the rim of the orbit, not against the eyeball!

Holding the eye open like this for more than a minute may become uncomfortable for the patient because the tear film is not being regenerated. This causes the surface of the eye to become dry and uncomfortable. People who cannot blink or close the eye report pain in the eye.

The Conjunctiva and Sclera

The conjunctiva is examined for redness, hemorrhages, abnormal pigmentation, or coloration. Pallor of the conjunctiva, especially the lower cul-de-sac, may indicate anemia or the reaction to a vasoconstrictor, such as sympathetic type eye dilating drops. (A possible cause is over-the-counter eye drops to "get the red out.") Dilated veins in the absence of inflammation, tearing, or pus may indicate congestive heart failure or an intracranial arterial-venous shunt, resulting in high venous pressure.

The apparent color of the conjunctiva is actually the color of the sclera as seen through the clear conjunctiva. Patients with dark skin color may have scattered dark pigmentation spots on the conjunctiva, especially near the edge of the cornea (the limbus). Yellow sclera may indicate jaundice from liver disease or massive hemolysis, while orange sclera is present in hypervitaminosis A (from the popular carrot juice diet). Blue sclera is seen in some collagen vascular diseases, like osteogenesis imperfecta, and in people who have received silver injections (used in the past to prevent polio). Pigmented spots are usually benign nevi but can be melanoma. The size of nevi should be recorded and followed for color change or growth that might indicate transformation into a melanoma.

Pink or yellow, raised fleshy areas of the conjunctiva between the eyelids when the eye is open may occur on the nasal or temporal side of the cornea. They are triangular in shape but are two different lesions. If the triangle points away from the cornea with the base of the triangle along the edge of the cornea but not involving the cornea, it is a pinguecula. It is caused by damage to the conjunctiva from sunlight or drying and represents a degeneration of the conjunctiva. They are only of cosmetic importance. If they grow, they may have become cancerous.

If the triangle is based in the conjunctiva away from the cornea and the apex points toward the cornea, usually onto the cornea, it is a pterygium. The pterygium is an attempt to heal actinic damage of the cornea. Conjunctiva migrates onto the cornea to cover the damage. The elevated pterygium lifts the tear spreading eyelid, causing drying and damage of the adjacent cornea. The pterygium then migrates to cover this damage and if not stopped can chase itself across the cornea to the pupil to distort or block vision. Pterygia are surgically removed but often recur because of the damage to the cornea that was not removed. (There are many procedures to remove pterygia demonstrating that none work very well.)

Tiny, less than one millimeter, black or brown spots on the sclera that are located three to four millimeters from the edge of the cornea are normal. They are points where nerve loops emerge from the sclera and carry pigment from the ciliary body. They can be a pathway for extension of intraocular melanoma, but this is very rare. These spots are called Axenfeld' loops and are identified by their location. They do not change. Spots that change color or size should raise suspicion of melanoma.

The lower conjunctiva should form a smooth cul-de-sac where it reflects from the eyelid to the sclera. Conjunctiva should appear wet and shiny. Dullness indicates a dry eye, possibly from vitamin A deficiency. The dry eye may be related to collagen vascular disease, especially rheumatoid disease, or the sequel to a chemical burn. It may be from scarring after Stevens-Johnson syndrome or benign mucus membrane pemphigoid, which destroys or occludes the tear glands and ducts.

The nasal corner of the eyelid opening should contain a pink mound of tissue, the caruncle, and a fold of conjunctiva, the plica semilunaris, between the caruncle and the conjunctiva that covers the sclera. These should both be smooth and shiny. Loss of definition of these structures, into a scar, is one of the first signs of benign ocular cicatricial pemphigoid (OCP).

Cornea

The cornea should appear wet and shiny and should be crystal clear. People with high cholesterol may have a white deposit ring in the peripheral one to two millimeters of the cornea called arcus senilis. There is usually a lucid space between the ring and the edge of the sclera. Older patients may have this white ring that contains metabolic debris from the cornea.

A copper colored band (brown or dark green) in the deep layers of the peripheral cornea, called a Kayser-Fleischer ring, may indicate Wilson disease, a copper storage disease affecting the brain, liver, and other organs. This ring is considered pathognomonic for Wilson disease. It may be seen with the naked eye, but it is best seen with the slit lamp. This disease usually presents with neurologic and psychiatric symptoms, but may present as liver or kidney failure.

Any opacity of the cornea may indicate scaring from prior injury or ulcers or may be active infectious disease. There are several corneal dystrophies that are characterized by grey or white deposits in the cornea or corneal edema that creates haze.

Corneal abrasions may be invisible to the naked eye, but may be detected in patients with light colored irises by moving the penlight back and forth and watching for a moving shadow on the iris from light refraction from the edge of the epithelium around the abrasion. Fluorescein eye drops will stain the denuded cornea, but not intact epithelium, to identify an abrasion.

The Iris

Using the penlight for illumination, inspect the surface of the iris. The iris should appear lacy and have a peripheral part that is thicker than the central portion. The central edge of the thicken part is called the collaret. The posterior pigment layer of the iris may be visible around the pupil edge as a thin rim of darker tissue. In diabetes, this rim may be wider and extend onto the front surface of the iris because of fibrovascular membrane formation that pulls the pigmented layer from behind the iris onto the anterior surface.

Because the iris is heavily pigmented on the posterior surface, it may have nevi, which appear as brown or black spots on the anterior surface. The pigment layers of the iris and ciliary body may give rise to melanomas. A ciliary body melanoma may cause the iris in that eye to become generally darker than the iris in the other eye, or only locally darker, over the tumor, or it may cause local displacement of the iris toward the cornea.

Heterochromia of the iris, or the difference of the color of the irises in the two eyes, may be normal or indicate pathology in either the lighter eye or the darker eye. The iris is usually lighter in color in the eye affected by a congenital Horner's syndrome (damage to the cervical sympathetic nervous system in the neck, oculosympathetic palsy, sometimes from birth trauma). The pupil is usually smaller on the effected side and the eyelid may droop (ptosis). Heterochromia, when part of the iris in one eye is darker that the rest of the iris, should indicate need for further evaluation for pathology, particularly melanoma. Uveitis in one eye may cause the iris in that eye to become darker.

The Crystalline Lens

The lens in the eye can be partially evaluated using the penlight without dilating the pupil. In an infant, the pupil should be completely black, but in most adults, the anterior surface of the lens can be seen just behind the pupil when illuminated from off center. It should be smooth and only faintly translucent.

Holding the penlight next to the examiners temple while shining it into the pupil will cause the light to reflect from the retina and make the pupil glow orange to red. (This is the red pupil seen in flash pictures caused by the flash being too close to the camera.) Any opacity between the retina and the examiners eye will be silhouetted against this red glow. By moving from right to left and back while observing the opacity, it can be determined whether the opacity is in front of the pupil or behind it. If the opacity moved the same direction in the pupil as the examiner is moving, it is behind the pupil. If it moves the opposite direction, the opacity is in front of the pupil. The extent of the movement is greater the farther the opacity is from the plane of the iris. An estimate can be made whether it is in the lens or vitreous behind the pupil or in the anterior chamber or cornea, in front of the iris.

The clarity of the lens can be judged by the brightness of the red reflex. As a cataract increases in density, the reflex becomes more orange and less bright. A dense senile cataract is white or yellow-brown. A posterior subcapsular cataract may appear as a fuzzy spot in the center of the red pupil or it may totally occlude the pupil. Congenital cataracts may appear as rings or spokes in the reflection.

If the pupil is dilated or mid-dilated, the position of the lens can be evaluated by looking for the edge of the lens, which is normally not seen. The lens should be centered behind the pupil. If it is displaced from this location, the edge of the lens may become visible at one edge of the pupil. A dislocated lens may indicate Marfan syndrome (arachnodactyly, high arched palate, and cardiac disease) or Weill-Marchesani syndrome (congenital mesodermal dysmorphodystrophy). The other common cause for dislocation of the lens is trauma to the eye or head. For more detailed examination of the lens, see the chapter on the Slit Lamp.

> In some parts of the world, cataracts are treated by inserting a needle into the eye and intentionally dislocating the lens back into the vitreous to clear the pupil. If the lens is broken in the process, it will cause significant uveitis resulting in blindness.

This is the extent of the routine examination of the eye using a penlight. Use of the penlight in a poor man's indirect ophthalmoscope will be discussed in a later chapter.

The penlight exam should not take more than two minutes if no pathology is present.

# Eyelids: Pathology and Detailed Exam

## Anatomy

The eyelids are composed of thin skin, which covers a cartilaginous plate (tarsal plate) in both upper and lower eyelids plus the circular orbicularis muscles. The backside of the tarsal plate is covered by conjunctiva. The leading edge of the eyelid, where upper and lower eyelids meet, is flat with square front and back edges and a faint grey line half way between the inner and outer surfaces. This line indicates where the skin of the outside of the eyelids transitions into the mucosa of the conjunctiva from the back of the eyelid.

There is a row of twenty to thirty glandular openings along this grey line in each eyelid. These are the openings of the meibomian glands that extend into the tarsal plate. Eyelashes emerge from the outer edge of the eyelid, anterior to the grey line, where the skin of the front of the eyelid bends over onto the edge of the eyelid. The hair follicles contain oil secreting glands called the glands of Moll.

The skin of the upper eyelid normally has a crease, parallel to the edge of the eyelid, about four or five millimeters from the edge of the eyelid. This crease indicates the upper edge of the tarsal plate where the skin is not held by the plate.

## Examination

The first level of the eye examination begins with the eyelids. Careful inspection will determine if the eyelids are symmetrical in size and shape. When the eyes are open, the upper eyelid should have a line or crease that demarcates the upper edge of the tarsal plate. The eyelid skin is firmly attached to the tarsal plate so it does not fold when the eyelid opens and closes. The skin above the tarsus folds to allow movement of the eyelid during blinking and movement of the eye. The tarsal plate in the lower eyelid is smaller and does not usually create a fold in the lower eyelid, which moves very little during blinking. When there is excess skin in the lower eyelids forming bags, the upper extent of the loose skin is at the lower edge of the tarsal plate of the lower eyelid.

The upper eyelid fold is created by the retraction of the upper eyelid by the levator muscle, which inserts into the upper edge of the tarsal plate. When the levator muscle is paralyzed or chronically ineffective at raising the eyelid, there is often no fold in the upper eyelid. Total absence of an eyelid fold usually accompanies congenital drooping of the eyelid called ptosis. Ptosis may occur in one or both eyes.

If there is some function in the levator muscle, the lid fissure width may vary when the patient is asked to look up or down. If ptosis is found, the lid fissure width of each eye should be measured (with a handy millimeter ruler) in up, down, and straight ahead gaze to determine the amount of levator function that exists.

Ptosis in a child may be severe enough that the eyelid covers the pupil, blocking vision. When this happens in one eye, that eye will usually develop amblyopia (lazy eye). This should be treated at an early age. When severe ptosis occurs in both eyes, the patient develops a head tilt, bending the head backward while looking down, beneath the drooping eyelids, to see ahead.

Chronic edema from allergies and skin laxity from aging may cause the skin to relax, stretching the upper eyelid. The skin may roll down over the front of the eyelid and press down on the eyelashes and weigh down the upper eyelid. This is called blepharochalasis. The skin may sag to the extent that it blocks the upper visual field. If visual field blockage is significant, surgical excision of the excess skin is indicated.

There are racial differences in the shape and position of the eyelids. Oriental people may have a band of skin in the nasal upper eyelid called an epiblepharon, causing the eye opening to have an almond shape. Non-oriental infants and small children may have this skin fold in the nasal upper eyelid that is lax skin caused by the delayed formation of the bridge of the nose. As the child grows and the nose develops, the extra skin is pulled away from the eye to cover the nose, causing the fold to disappear.

The edges of the eyelids should be smooth with the upper and lower eyelids well opposed when closed. Each eyelid had two regions. There is a short section at the nasal end of the eyelid. This ends at the lacrimal punctum, a small hole in the eyelid margin with slightly raised edge. The lacrimal canaliculus runs from this hole to the lacrimal sac, which is located behind the ligaments extending from the nasal ends of the eyelids to the medial wall of the orbit, and extends into the lower nasal quadrant of the eye socket (orbit). There is a canaliculus in each eyelid, upper and lower.

The eyelid edge from the punctum to the temporal end of the eyelid contains the lashes and glands and should be well opposed to the eyeballs along the entire length. Aging, chronic allergy, and or trauma may cause the lower eyelid to sag away from the eyeball, leaving an open sac of conjunctiva exposed to the air. This condition is called lagophthalmos.

When the eyelid is not opposed to the eyeball, the tears will rundown into the open sac to flow onto the cheek. Tears do not spread over the eyeball with blinking, resulting in drying of the ocular surface.

This sagging skin may be caused by excess skin and swelling below the eye called dermatochalasis, or by laxity of the ligaments that hold the ends of the tarsal plates to the orbital rim. Pulling up and out on the temporal end of the lower eyelid should bring the edge of the eyelid into opposition with the eyeball. If the eyelid does not move up toward the eyeball, there is probably scarring in the skin or subcutaneous tissues of the lower eyelid holding it down. There are several surgical procedures designed to correct lagophthalmos.

Relaxation of the skin of the eyelids may cause bags under the eyes. This is often accompanied by breaks in the orbital septum that allow orbital fat to herniate through the septum to fill the bags of excess skin. Looseness of the skin of the upper eyelid such that it hangs over the lashes can obstruct the upper field of vision. Breaks in the orbital septum allow orbital fat to herniate from the orbit into the subcutaneous tissues increasing the size of the bags and causing bulges in the upper eyelids also, especially nasally.

The eyelashes should be uniformly distributed along the eyelid margin and be uniform in color and length. When lashes fall out, leaving gaps, it is called madarosis. This is indicative of an underlying disease, such as blepharitis, or a generalized skin disease. Lashes usually do not grow in cancers, such as squamous cell or basal cell tumors of the eyelid margins. Madarosis of the eyelids and eyebrows also occurs in leprosy. (Detailed examination of the lashes will be covered further in the Slit Lamp Examination chapter.)

The eyebrows are usually positioned along the upper rim of the eye socket (orbit). Normally the skin between the eyebrows above the nose, called the glabella, is hairless. In some patients, brows may extend nasally to form a continuous line of hair, or a unibrow. The hair of the eyebrows should be uniform in color and length, although grooming habits, like eyebrow plucking and dyeing, may cause changes in the distribution and coloration of the hair.

Aging of the skin of the forehead or the onset of a facial palsy may cause the eye brow to sag below the orbital rim and allow the skin of the upper eyelid to sag down upon the lashes and hang over the visual pathway. Aging involves both sides of the face, but Bell's palsy usually only affects one side. Depending upon the cause of the Bell's palsy, nerve function may return after regeneration of the nerve. If the brow ptosis is severe, the hair of a bushy eyebrow may scratch the cornea. This can be treated by trimming of the eyebrows. There are several approaches to surgical correction of brow ptosis, if it is considered permanent.

Diseases like trachoma, ocular cicatricial pemphigoid, severe chemical burn of the eye, or Stevens-Johnson syndrome may cause scarring of the posterior side of the eyelid. This may pull the edge of the eyelid posteriorly, causing the lashes to rub the cornea. Individual lashes may grow in an errant manor and emerge from the posterior edge of the eyelid to rub the cornea. This is call trichiasis. To determine the cause of trichiasis involving the upper eyelid, it is necessary to evert the upper eyelid.

Eversion of the Upper Eyelid

Eversion of the eyelid is easily accomplished using the stick end of a cotton-tipped applicator (the cotton ball end is too large) or a small- to medium-sized paperclip that is bent open into a flat figure eight. The lower half of the upper eyelid is rigid because of the tarsal plate. The upper edge of the tarsal plate is demarcated by the first skin fold above the lid margin (about three to five millimeters above the lash line).

The patient is asked to look down. This relaxes the levator muscle, which actively opposes the eversion maneuver if the patient looks straight ahead.

With the hand closest to the patient's nose, grasp the eyelashes of the lid to be everted with the thumb and index finger (the more lashes the better). Pull down and out on the lashes, releasing the suction between the eyeball and eyelid while placing the stick or paperclip just above the lid fold to hold it in position. (Do not press down or against the eyeball.) Pull the lashes upward, flipping the tarsal plate back on the eyelid around the stick or paper clip. By maintaining pressure on the eyelashes against the orbital rim, the underside of the eyelid may be examined. The patient must continue to look down. After examining the conjunctiva, having the patient look up will reposition the eyelid.

This is a useful maneuver to perform when the patient complains of a foreign body sensation in the eye and no foreign body can be seen on the surface of the eye. Foreign bodies can become embedded in the conjunctiva covering the tarsal plate. They rub the cornea with each blink and, if found, must be removed with a cotton tipped applicator or the tip of a small needle mounted on an insulin syringe or cotton-tipped applicator. It is best to instill topical anesthesia in the eye before removing a foreign body (i.e., before everting the eyelid).

To examine the entire upper conjunctival cul-de-sac it is necessary to double evert the upper eyelid. This can be done by using a flat stent, such as the paperclip, or a microbiology spatula, in the procedure above. Once the lid is everted, the paperclip is rotated a half turn (90°, not 180°), producing another partial fold of the eyelid that pulls the upper conjunctiva in to the field of vision. This is useful in looking for lost contact lenses when the patient feels that the contact lens in still in the eye and has slid into the upper fornix.

Whereas the single eversion of the eyelid is not very uncomfortable, double eversion is definitely uncomfortable and should be done briefly, only when indicated and usually with the benefit of topical anesthesia.

Eyelid Position, Shape, and Movement

Ptosis can be congenital or acquired. The difference is determined by history. The upper eyelid skin in congenital ptosis does not show a skin fold in the upper eyelid. Acquired ptosis can be from trauma to the levator nerve, cranial third nerve disease or injury, or excessive eye rubbing.

A history of a droopy eyelid that occurs in one eye on some days and the other eye on other days should immediately suggest myasthenia. To bring this out, the examination is directed toward fatiguing the neuromuscular junction. To do this, the patient is asked to look up at an object in the examiners hand and hold the vision on the object. In muscular dystrophy, the upper eyelid will fatigue and drift downward to cover the pupil. This can also be demonstrated by having the patient follow an object up and down repeatedly. The lid will begin to fatigue and not be able to go all the way up after several up and down swings. The function should recover in a few minutes.

Ptosis from myasthenia may be accompanied by ocular muscle imbalance in one or more extra-ocular muscles, causing double vision. If suspected, this should be looked for and brought out by repetitive eye movements, following an object back and forth in the active fields of the various muscles. Myasthenia can occur in only the eyes or may be combined with the systemic disease. Systemic myasthenia may present in the eyes and later spread to the remainder of the body.

Other forms of lid anomalies include entropion, the inward turning of the eyelid that causes the eyelashes to rub the cornea, and ectropion, the outward turning or sagging of the eyelid.

Spastic entropion is common in older patients who have laxity of the skin and eyelids. The lashes irritate the conjunctiva and cornea, causing the patient to squeeze the eye, folding the lid margin into the eye. Gentle retraction of the lower eyelid will evert the eyelid. It will stay in position until the patient squeezed the eye again. It is a repeating cycle of irritation and closure, causing entropion.

Children may be born with abnormally increased distance between the nasal ends of the eyelids. This distance should be approximately equal to the length of one horizontal eyelid opening. This horizontal displacement is known as telecanthus. This is often accompanied by short lid fissures with or without ptosis called blepharophimosis. A congenital midface anomaly may occur with ptosis, blepharophimosis, telecanthus, and poorly developed nose.

The skin of the eyelids is loosely attached to the underlying muscles allowing eyelid movement. This looseness allows for rapid swelling or infiltration beneath the skin. Edema fluid from trauma, allergic reactions, renal failure, or heart disease may collect around the eyes. In hypothyroid disease, the edema is from infiltration of mucopolysaccharides, so it is doughy and may pit with finger pressure.

The eyelids are a frequent site of skin cancers. The skin of the eyelids must be carefully examined for squamous cell and basal cell cancers. These occur commonly in the nasal end of the eyelids, but they can involve the lid margins or the thin skin of the upper or lower eyelids. Basal cell carcinoma presents as an elevated mass with a depression in the center. The edges can be described as pearl-like in appearance. Basal cell tumors may invade adjacent tissue, but tend to metastasize late.

Squamous carcinoma presents as an elevated mass of uniform consistency, usually attached to underlying tissue. It may have an identifiable blood supply. Squamous cell tumors may metastasize early.

Neuromas from neurofibromatosis (von Recklinghausen's disease) frequently occur on the face and eyelids. These may be associated with gliomas and meningiomas. Von Recklinghausen's disease also has characteristic pigmented skin lesions.

Any pigmented area should be examined for solid tumor, satellite pigmented spots, or tumor fixed to underlying tissue, with melanoma in mind. Some patients may have multiple skin cancers of the eyelids, especially those with xeroderma pigmentosum.

Patients with high cholesterol may have xanthelasma (i.e., small round white or yellow deposits in the skin of the nasal ends of the upper and lower eyelids). These spots may coalesce. These can be removed surgically for cosmetic reasons, but often recur if the blood cholesterol levels are not lowered.

Examination of the eyelids is not complete without examination of the meibomian gland orifices. Redness around the orifices, dandruff-like flakes among the lashes, and sleeves or nits on the lashes may indicate bacterial invasion or louse infestation of the meibomian glands. Light pressure on the lower eyelid just below the lash line may cause expression of clear or hazy oil from the glands. Hazy oil indicates inflammation, possibly bacterial. Chronic blepharitis may cause thickened secretions that extrude from the gland orifice like toothpaste from the tube, when light pressure is applied to the skin near the lash line. Thick secretions that are bluish-green in color may indicate pseudomonas blepharitis. This is not uncommon in immune suppressed patients (e.g., chemotherapy or AIDS patients).

Blockage of one or more of the meibomian glands of the eyelid margin may cause local swelling in the tarsal plate area of the eyelid. This may be red and tender to touch. It is called a chalazion. They may be infected or sterile. The lay term for this is an eyelid cyst.

Swelling of the eyelid margin around a hair follicle that distorts the eyelid margin around the hair follicle orifice, often with a central white spot, is called a hordeolum, or sty. This is an abscess of a gland of Moll. Most ophthalmologists advise against squeezing these to pop them because the pressure may spread the infection. (Cavernous sinus thrombosis, or sepsis, may result.) Warm compresses will cause the abscess to localize, point, and drain, relieving the problem. Some ophthalmologists will use a sterile needle to puncture and drain the hordeolum, but this is not recommended. Most physicians are not comfortable with sharp needles around the eye.

The External Eyeball (Front Surface)

When the eyelids are open, part of the front of the eyeball is visible. The white part that is visible is the sclera, seen through the clear conjunctiva. The sclera is composed of collagen fibers that are woven together randomly. This makes the sclera opaque to slightly translucent.

Beneath the sclera, there is a pigmented tissue, the choroid that further blocks light from entering the eye. The sclera is usually thick enough that the darker layer is not visible, so the sclera appears snow white.

There may be several small black dots in the sclera that are located several millimeters from the edge of the cornea. These are caused by nerve loops that come to the surface from beneath the sclera and double back immediately. Pigment follows these nerves and is visible from the surface. These spots may be very sensitive to touch. They are called Axenfeld loops.

When one or more localized blue spots of varying size and shape can be seen in the anterior sclera, they are usually caused by erosion of the sclera by rheumatoid disease. The sclera becomes very thin or perforates, allowing the underlying blue-black choroid tissue to protrude beneath the conjunctiva in a condition known as scleromalacia or, if through the entire thickness of the sclera, scleromalacia perforans. Pressure on the eye may cause the choroid to perforate beneath the conjunctiva, so do not press on the eye.

There may be scattered pigment on the surface of the sclera. Pigmented plaques are called nevi. Darkly pigmented races may have more nevi on the sclera. The most common site of these is the temporal sclera where it is exposed to light when the eye is open.

In infants, the sclera is often very thin and the underlying pigmented tissues show through, giving the sclera a blue tint. This disappears with time. Older children with persistent blue sclera may have a collagen disease like osteogenesis imperfecti.

Two diseases may cause the sclera to appear yellow or orange. These are 1) jaundice from liver disease, gall bladder obstruction, or hemolysis, causing bilirubin absorption in the sclera; and 2) vitamin A excess from high carotene diets that leads to carotene accumulation in the sclera. In vitamin A excess, the palms and soles are often orange with thickened and cracked skin.

The extraocular muscles attach to the sclera from five to seven millimeters from the edge of the cornea, but the muscles are covered by ligaments and fascia and not usually visible on examination.

There are vessels imbedded within the sclera, which are not usually visible. These vessels coalesce in a vascular network that encircles the anterior edge of the sclera where it meets the cornea. When there is inflammation within the eyeball or injury to the cornea, these vessels dilate, causing a pink or red ring around the cornea. This is called ciliary flush and usually indicates a serious problem within the eye or involving the cornea.

The sclera is covered with a layer of tissue called the conjunctiva. The conjunctiva covers the back surface of the eyelids and the surface of the eyeball, except for the surface of the cornea. This tissue consists of an epithelial layer, which is held on the eyelids and sclera by a loose connective tissue. This connective tissue is firmly adherent to the back of the eyelids, but very loosely connected to the eyeball and the zone of reflection where it passes from the eyelids to the eyeball. This allows very free movement of the eyeball.

The anterior edge of the conjunctiva, where it meets the cornea, is fused to the sclera at the limbus. The conjunctival epithelium undergoes a transition to corneal epithelium. The conjunctival epithelium contains goblet cells that secrete mucin, small lacrimal glands that produce tears, and white blood cells to combat disease. The corneal epithelium is devoid of these glands and white blood cells.

There are two special structures of the conjunctiva in the nasal corner of the eye: the caruncle and the semilunar fold, also called the plica semilunaris. The caruncle is a pink mound of tissue behind the nasal end of the eyelids. It fills the void between the eyelids when the eyes are open. Next to the caruncle there is a one millimeter wide fold of conjunctiva between the caruncle and the cornea. There is a small pocket or cul-de-sac behind the fold, which is a potential space. Scarring of the conjunctiva from chemical burns or trauma in the nasal conjunctiva may obliterate the caruncle and semilunar fold. In the absence of burns or trauma, fusion of the caruncle and semilunar fold into an ill-defined mass usually indicates ocular cicatricial pemphigoid—an autoimmune disease that causes shrinkage of the conjunctiva, symblepharon (adhesions between the eyelids and the eyeball), dry eye, ulceration, and scarring that can lead to blindness.

The refection of the conjunctiva from the back surface of the eyelids onto the surface of the eyeball creates a pocket or cul-de-sac behind the upper and lower eyelids and also temporally along the side of the eye. These cul-de-sacs allow the eye to move freely. The mucus and tear glands supply the lubrication to allow the conjunctiva to slide over itself without friction. The conjunctival epithelium continues the epithelial barrier of the body from the edges of the eyelid skin to cover the eye. The epithelium of the cornea completes the barrier. The conjunctival tissues contain a multitude of protective functions. The conjunctival tissue at the edge of the cornea contains stem cells to repair damage to the conjunctiva and cornea.

The conjunctiva has a rich blood supply with some vessels visible on inspection. Dilation of these vessels causes the conjunctiva to appear pink or red. The location of the redness may indicate an area of trauma or foreign body. The redness may localize to only the limbus adjacent to a corneal foreign body. Conjunctival injection or redness is usually diffuse in the area of injury, while ciliary flush from sclera vessels is located within two or three millimeters of the cornea.

Hemorrhages beneath the conjunctiva are usually bright red. They may spread beneath the conjunctiva and around the cornea. The most significant cause of sub-conjunctival hemorrhage is vascular hypertension. These hemorrhages occur spontaneously and may occur in both eyes.

More common causes include coughing, sneezing, and the Valsalva maneuver from straining (lifting or constipation) or vomiting. The seriousness of these is determined by the cause of each. Subconjunctival hemorrhages from causes other than hypertension can be simply observed as they change color and reabsorb over the next several days to a week.

Pigmented nevi may occur in the conjunctiva. It is important to determine whether the nevus is freely movable with the conjunctiva over the sclera. A nevus attached to the sclera may be an invasive melanoma. The surface of the eye is anesthetized with topical drops before trying to move the suspected lesion over the underlying tissue with a cotton tipped applicator.

Blue-black pigmentation of the skin over the distribution of branches one and two of the fifth cranial nerve and conjunctiva on one side of the face may be a Nevus of Ota. This pigmentation may involve the iris and choroid within the eye. This lesion is usually benign, but may transform into a melanoma. This transformation occurs in about 4% of cases, so it must be watched for a change in shape or pigmentation, indicating a melanoma.

Cornea

Anatomy

The center of the front of the eyeball is a round clear window called the cornea. It is slightly more than a half millimeter thick in the center and almost a millimeter thick where it fuses with the sclera. The curvature of the cornea is slightly steeper than the sclera, so the central cornea protrudes above the imaginary surface of the sclera sphere. The cornea is like the crystal of a wristwatch. The zone where the cornea fuses into the sclera is called the limbus. The limbus is where the curvature changes and coincides with the edge of the white sclera.

The cornea is composed of five distinct layers. The outermost layer is the epithelium, which is made of cells. The cells closest to the basement membrane to which it is attached are tightly packed columnar cells. As these reproduce, the cells are pushed outward and become wing shaped layers. As they mature, they become flattened squamous cells. The sixth and seventh layers slough off into the tear film.

The second layer of the cornea is a tightly packed layer of interwoven collagen fibers with mucopolysaccharide filler. This is called Bowman's layer. Behind Bowman's layer is a thick layer of more loosely woven collagen fibers with a mucopolysaccharide filler called the stroma. Behind this stroma is a strong clear membrane called Descemet's membrane that serves as basement membrane for the corneal endothelium. The endothelium that lines the back of Descemet's membrane is a one cell thick layer of tightly bound hexagonal cells.

The epithelium is constantly being replaced by new cells and has the ability to detach from the basement membrane and migrate to close gaps created by trauma or disease. Epithelium continues to grow and repair throughout life.

The endothelium cells continue to reproduce until a child is about two years old. At that point, no more cells are produced, so it must heal by sliding and thinning. If the endothelium thins too much, it can no longer perform its main function of limiting the flow of aqueous humor into the cornea and pumping fluid from the cornea, so edema ensues.

The cornea is clear because it contains glycosaminoglycans (mucopolysaccharides) between the collagen fibers that give the cornea its structural strength. Sclera does not have these glycosaminoglycans, so it is opaque.

> This difference can be demonstrated by soaking a Millipore filter in alcohol and holding it in the light path from a projector. The alcohol soaked filter will allow the light to pass through the filter to project a sharp image. As the alcohol evaporates, the filter becomes more opaque, eventually blocking the light from the projector.

The cornea should be clear, smooth, and shiny and have a luster. A dull cornea is dry or has some opacity or surface problem. The anterior surface of the cornea is the first optical surface encountered by light entering the eye where the cornea begins the focusing process. This surface is very important. The cornea is covered with an epithelial layer that is several cell layers thick, but uneven. This slightly irregular surface is covered by a layer of tears. Damage to this epithelial layer, the tear film, or edema of the cells may disrupt vision significantly.

Examination

Using a penlight to illuminate the front of the eye, the examiner should see a single spot of light reflection on the cornea. Multiple spot reflections indicate roughness, distortion, or corneal edema with bullae (tiny edema blisters within the epithelium). Edema of the cornea may also cause a central grey-white haze, especially if the penlight is shown on the cornea from the side.

Old ulcers or trauma may leave opaque scars on the cornea, which appear grey or white. Old scars may vascularize with visible blood vessels. These vessels may become empty potential vessels, which are usually invisible unless seen as cellophane wrinkles against the reflected light from the iris. With trauma or infection, these vessels become filled with blood, indicating active disease.

Holding a penlight very close to the axis of the eye while looking into the eye should cause the red light reflex. This is when the light entering the eye is reflected from the retina, causing red light to fill the pupil. Any opacity of the cornea, lens, or vitreous in the path of the light will be silhouetted against this light. Movement of the examiner, or the examined eye, from side to side will determine whether the opacity is in front of the pupil or behind it. The eye can be moved by the examiner holding up a finger in front of the patient and moving it side to side while the patient is watching the finger. The examiner views the red pupil as the eye moves.

Patients with high cholesterol or older patients may have a white deposit in the peripheral cornea near the edge of the cornea, usually forming a complete circle. This is called arcus senilis. In older patients, it is from a degenerative process and is of no significance except cosmetic. In young patients, it may be cholesterol deposits, so it should prompt a serum lipid evaluation.

The curvature of the cornea is critical in focusing light on the retina. Flatter corneas do not bend the light enough to focus it on the retina, causing hyperopia, (farsightedness), while steep corneas bend the light too much, resulting in myopia, (nearsightedness). Symmetrically curved or warped corneas cause distortion in light focusing called regular astigmatism. The variations in corneal curvature that cause these errors in the refraction of light are usually too subtle to be determined by observation. They can be determined by optical measurement of light refraction as in fitting glasses by measurement of ring reflection with the keratoscope, or by computerized analysis of light reflection from the cornea.

In keratoconus, a disease of ectasia (i.e., thinning of the cornea), the cornea may visibly bulge forward. This can be demonstrated by having the patient look down so that the central cornea is against the edge of the lower eyelid. The distortion of the lower eyelid by the bulging cornea will be more obvious. This is called Munson's sign. Keratoconus is a primary disease, but it also occurs in patients with other eye diseases. It is associated with Down's syndrome, atopic dermatitis, Marfan syndrome, and Ehlers-Danlos syndrome.

Sensation of the cornea is through the fifth cranial nerve (CN V). Damage to this nerve may cause partial or total loss of sensation. Prolonged contact lens wear (for months) may decrease the sensitivity of the corneal nerves. Diseases like herpes simplex or zoster and leprosy permanently damage the nerves and numb the cornea. Diabetic damage to the fifth cranial nerve also decreases corneal sensation.

Testing for corneal sensation is usually done with a cotton wisp or piece of dental floss. A wisp of cotton can be teased from a cotton-tipped applicator to form a thin fiber extending from the applicator. This wisp is brought in from the side of the patient's face to touch the central cornea. This should elicit a reflex blink or head jerk away from the fiber. If the wisp can touch the cornea and rest on the cornea without a response, the nerve is significantly damaged. The patient should be asked whether they can feel the wisp and how the two eyes compare.

Careful examination of the cornea may reveal pigmented lines on the surface. A circular brown line around the central cornea, called a Kayser-Fleischer ring, may demarcate the edge of the central cone of keratoconus. A horizontal brown line (iron deposits) across the lower cornea is called a Hudson-Stahli line. The brown line around the leading edge of a pterygium is called a Stocker's line. These lines usually do not affect vision.

Lines and shapes may develop on the posterior surface of the cornea that can best be seen in retro-illumination of the cornea. A brown spindle shaped area on the back of the cornea may be seen normally in young pregnant women and in pigmentary glaucoma.

White blood cells may accumulate in a triangle on the back of the lower cornea in patients with intraocular inflammation. The apex on the triangle is at the center of the cornea. This is caused by precipitation of the white cells as they circulate within the anterior chamber. The iris is warm, so the aqueous containing the cells in front of the iris moves upward. The cornea is cooler so the aqueous, containing the cells, cools, and falls, causing the cells to be caught on the lower cornea as it recedes toward the limbus. The aqueous also has a split circulation away from the center of the cornea as it descends, leading to the triangular shape of the deposit.

This white triangle is not the same as a flat-topped layer of white cells that accumulates between the iris and the back of the cornea.

This layer is the result of inflammation from bacterial infection or uveitis. This layer is called a hypopyon and indicates severe or chronic inflammation.

The cornea is subject to congenital dystrophies that cause metabolites to accumulate in various layers of the cornea. These may be seen a tiny opacities or roughness of the surface. The shape of the opacities and their distribution determine the name of the dystrophy and the progression and type of visual loss to be expected. Macular dystrophy has many little fuzzy spots that cause loss of vision, whereas granular dystrophy has sharp edged spots with clear cornea between, delaying visual loss. There are many named dystrophies characterized by the shape and location of the opacities.

Fuch' dystrophy involves the corneal endothelium caused by excrescences on Descemet's membrane that stretch and interrupt the endothelium, causing it to leak, creating corneal edema. This endothelial damage is not seen with the naked eye. The edema can be seen as haziness of the corneal epithelium and micro blisters within the epithelium. These produce an etched glass appearance to the central cornea, which appears grey or white by penlight illumination.

The Lacrimal System

The front of the eye is bathed in a layer of tears to make the surface optically smooth and keep it wet. Most ophthalmologists consider the tear film a sixth and anterior most layer of the cornea because tears are so related to the function of the cornea. The surface of the cornea is microscopically rough. The tears cover the roughness to create an optically smooth surface.

There are three components to the tear film. The major component of tears is water from the lacrimal glands. The posterior layer is composed of mucin from the goblet cells of the conjunctiva. Mucin is rubbed onto the cornea by the eyelids during blinking. Mucin makes the surface of the eye hydrophilic, allowing the water component of the tear film to spread over the cornea and conjunctiva. The outer layer of the tear film is a thin coating of oils from the meibomian glands of the eyelid margin. The oil retards evaporation and stabilizes the tear film.

Some of the watery component of tears is produced by the main lacrimal gland, which resides in the upper temporal quadrant of the orbit (eye socket). This gland is connected through the orbital septum to the upper conjunctival cul-de-sac by four to eight ducts. There are also many tiny tear glands embedded in the conjunctiva. These tiny glands are responsible for maintenance level tearing while the main lacrimal gland turns on and off on demand in response to irritation, dryness, and emotions.

When adequate tears are present, they pool along the lower eyelid where it rests against the eyeball. Close examination will reveal a meniscus of tears along the lower eyelid and ocular surface. Absence of this meniscus indicates a dry eye. The cause may be lack of watery tear production, excessive drying from wind or low humidity, or mechanical positioning of the lower eyelid, allowing the tears to flow behind the eyelid into the cul-de-sac or out of the eye or because of a decreased blinking rate due to thyroid disease.

After the tear film is spread over the cornea by the eyelid, the water portion may drain from between the mucus and oil layers, allowing these two layers to come in contact. This creates a dry spot on the cornea. These dry spots can best be visualized by putting Fluorescein in the tear film and watching with blue light for dark spots where the stain containing watery portion has disappeared. The time from opening the eye until the dry spots appear is called the tear film break up time or BUT. The duration for tear film breakup correlates with lack of water component—shorter breakup, less aqueous layer.

When the oil layer mixes with the mucus layer, it may form a thin film on the cornea. As the eyelids blink, this film is rolled into strands that float in the tear film and are moved toward the nasal end of the lid fissure by the eyelid blinking. The strands tend to curl into small mucus balls that collect in the corner of the eye. Patients may pull these strands from the eye and think they are tiny worms. Patients with mucus in the corner of the eye may have dry eyes or a blocked lacrimal canaliculus.

Another sign of a dry eye is the bunching of temporal conjunctiva along the temporal part of the lower eyelid. Since the conjunctiva is dry and not well lubricated, it does not slide behind the eyelid but bunches in tiny horizontal folds along the lid margin.

Excessive Tearing

A blocked canaliculus will prevent the tears from flowing into the lacrimal sac in the lower nasal orbit and then down into the nose. The canaliculi may be blocked by trauma, infection, or chronic use of certain ocular medications such as idoxuridine (IDU) for herpes simplex and certain glaucoma eye drops. A blocked tear duct will cause the tears to pool along the lower eyelid and blur vision. Excessive tearing, called epiphora, may also be caused paradoxically by a dry eye. The eye detects dryness and sporadically turns on the main lacrimal gland, which causes overflow tearing. This may be the first symptom of a dry eye.

The openings of the canaliculi are on the eyelid margin near the nasal end of the upper and lower eyelids. The hole in the lid margin, called the lacrimal punctum, is visible and should blend in with the surrounding color of the eyelid. If the edge of the hole is red or elevated, the canaliculus may be infected. The duct may also close because of normal aging and will need to be dilated or opened with various snip procedures.

The canaliculi run from the eyelid to the lacrimal sac, which is located behind the medial palpebral ligament that holds the eyelids to the nasal orbital wall. The sack extends down to the lacrimal fossa where it narrows to become the lacrimal duct, which empties the tears into the nose under the inferior nasal turbinate.

An ophthalmologist may place fluorescein in the tear film where the tears should carry it to the nose where it can be recovered by passing a cotton-tipped applicator into the nose beneath the inferior turbinate. Alternatively, if fluorescein is produced by blowing the nose, the cotton swab test is unnecessary. This is called the Jones I test. If no dye is found after five minutes, the canaliculus is dilated and probed with a punctal irrigating needle. Saline with fluorescein is gently irrigated into the sac and should flood the nose. If no fluid is passed into the nose, the system is blocked. The irrigation phase is called the Jones II test.

The lacrimal sac is usually not palpable in the lower nasal orbit unless it is obstructed or contains a tumor. A blocked lacrimal duct will cause the lacrimal sac to swell and overflow back through the canaliculi. Infection of the lacrimal sac may cause pronounced swelling and redness near the nose. Gentle pressure on the swollen area may cause extrusion of mucus and pus from the lacrimal puncta. Drainage must be established to cure this condition. Probing, after the infection is controlled by antibiotics, may open the duct to create drainage and allow the sac and duct to heal.

The most common test of tear function used by ophthalmologists is the Schirmer I test. Special strips of Whatman 41 filter paper, with a small notch near one end, are used to absorb the tears for a five minute period. The strips are bent at a right angle at the notch. The short end is placed behind the lower eye such that the notch is at the inner edge of the eyelid. The tears should wet at least five millimeters of the strip by five minutes as measured from the notch. Placing the strips into the eye without first anesthetizing the eye (classic Schirmer 1 test) may produce more tears by irritation. To avoid this, the eye can be anesthetized with eye drops and excess drops blotted from the cul-de-sac before the strips are placed. This is a better measure of baseline secretion, because it simulates the usual condition of the patient without external stimulation.

A measure of maximum tear production uses a cotton swab to irritate the nasal mucosa at the beginning of the test to determine the maximum tear output on the filter paper strips for five minutes. Normal production is greater than fifteen millimeters on the strip. This is called the Schirmer II test. It is used to diagnose severe failure of tear production.

The main lacrimal gland in the upper outer quadrant of the orbit is usually not visible or palpable. It may swell if infected by bacteria and during mumps.

Staining of the Dry Eye

Rose Bengal eye drops applied to a chronically dry eye will produce punctate staining of the area of the cornea and conjunctiva, which is normally exposed between the eyelids when the eye is open. This punctate staining can be graded by scoring the dots in four quadrants of the upper and lower nasal and temporal conjunctiva and cornea (5 areas) from 1+ to 3+ and adding the total score (0 to 15).

# Examination of the Inner Eye

The Direct Ophthalmoscope

The handheld direct ophthalmoscope is used to examine the retina and choroid through the pupil. It is called a direct ophthalmoscope because the examiner looks directly at the retina. (With the indirect ophthalmoscope, the examiner looks at a virtual image of the retina.)

The direct ophthalmoscope is a simple instrument that uses a light and mirror and a set of lenses to overcome the physical difficulties encountered when looking at the retina. To look into the eye, the examiner aligns their visual axis with that of the patient by looking through the pupil. The normal eye is focused at infinity with parallel rays entering the eye focused on the retina. The reflected light rays from the retina are optically aligned by the eyeball to be parallel as they emerge from the eye. If the viewing eye is focused at infinity, the intercepted light rays should focus on the viewer's retina. If either eye is not normally focused at infinity (i.e., nearsighted or farsighted), the image will not be in focus. The lenses in the ophthalmoscope within the viewing aperture are there to correct for this focusing problem. Simply click through the dial until the correct lens is in place to bring the retina into focus.

In order to align the optical axis of both the examinee and examiner and be close enough to see into the eye, the examiners head will block most of the available light that enters the eye being examined. To overcome this problem, a light bulb is placed in the head of the ophthalmoscope with the light beam directed into the eye by a mirror or prism. The viewing aperture is directly above the light source so that the light can be directed through the pupil and the examiner can look through the pupil down the beam of light.

The skill in using an ophthalmoscope is to shine the light through the lower half of the pupil while looking through the center or upper half of the pupil. Some of the light from the ophthalmoscope is usually reflected from the front surface of the cornea, causing glare at a brightness several log units more powerful than the light reflected from the retina. This glare obliterates the view of the retina. To avoid this glare, the light must enter the eye below the center of the pupil and center of the cornea. The curvature of the cornea will reflect the light away from the viewing aperture, allowing the retina to be seen.

The lens system of the ophthalmoscope varies with the manufacturer. Usually the lenses are in one diopter steps from -10 to +10, which allows good focus for the majority of patients. Patients who have had a cataract removed without an intraocular implant lens may require a +10 to +20 lenses. Some ophthalmoscopes have additional -10, +10, and/or +20 lenses that can be added to the single diopter step lenses to create a sharp focus.

Use of the Ophthalmoscope

The ease of using the direct ophthalmoscope to examine the retina depends to a large degree on the positioning of both the patient and the examiner. The preferred position is to have the patient seated on an elevated chair or an examination table, facing the examiner. The examiner stands or sits to the outside of the patient's knees.

Alternatively, the patient may be examined lying on an exam table, looking at the ceiling. The examiner bends over the patient from the side to be examined.

The patient is asked to look at a specific spot, straight ahead (e.g., a clock, a picture, a piece of tape on the wall, etc). Telling the patient to look straight ahead will not make them hold the eye steady. Looking at a specific object will keep the eye still.

When examining the patient's right eye, the examiner holds the ophthalmoscope in their right hand and looks through the aperture of the ophthalmoscope with the examiner's right eye. Then use the left hand and left eye when examining the patient's left eye.

Unless the patient has a scarred cornea, a dense cataract or some other intraocular opacity, the light does not have to be at full power. There is a rheostat on the ophthalmoscope to adjust the light. For patient cooperation, it is best to use the minimum amount of light to produce a good image of the retina while not temporarily blinding the patient.

The free hand is used to steady the patient and lift the upper eyelid. This is done by placing the fingers across the forehead above the eye and using the thumb to gently draw the loose skin of the eyelid up to the upper rim of the orbit. Gentle thumb pressure will hold the eye open without hurting the patient.

The examiner places the ophthalmoscope in front of their own eye when they are about ten inches from the patient. If possible, the examiner should keep both eyes open to avoid accommodation (focusing) with the examining eye. The ophthalmoscope is moved to direct the beam of light into the pupil. This should turn the pupil bright red. If the light is entering the pupil and the pupil is not red, there is a significant visual obstruction (corneal scar, hyphema, cataract, vitreous hemorrhage, or vitreous membrane) within the eye and the retina may not be visible.

The examiner moves toward the patient, keeping the pupil centered in their vision. This will bring the eyes into alignment and the retina should come into view. If there is glare, the examiner should lower the ophthalmoscope slightly (i.e., usually less than millimeter) until the glare is displaced away from the viewing aperture so the retina is visible. Tilting the ophthalmoscope a degree or two down will also change the angle of the reflected light away from the viewing aperture. Some ophthalmoscopes have a polarized filter to reduce glare. This filter may not be sufficient to remove all glare if the above technique is not followed.

At this point, the examiner is usually displaced temporally with respect to the optical axis of the patient. The patient should still be looking past the examiner at the spot on the wall, not at the examiner's light, and may need to be reminded to look at the spot. This temporal displacement of the examiner will usually cause the examiner to be looking at the nasal retina, at, or very close, to the optic nerve head. The optic nerve head is the best place to start the examination. If the nerve head is not within the viewing area, use the vessels to find it. The branches of the vessels form *V*s that point back along the vessels toward the nerve head.

Since there are no rods or cones on the nerve head, it is the visual blind spot, so the light will not bother the patient when most of the illuminated spot shines on the nerve head. By this same reasoning, it is best to save the examination of the very sensitive macula until last.

There are usually two or more spot sizes available on the ophthalmoscope. Use of the smaller spot is more comfortable for the patient. Large lesions of the retina may require the larger spot size.

To see into the eye, the ophthalmoscope should be within one half inch of the eye. To avoid bumping the eye and startling the patient, the examiner can rest the top of the ophthalmoscope against the thumb they are using to hold the upper eyelid. This does not bother the patient and saves embarrassment to the examiner by preventing the ophthalmoscope from touching the eye. It also gives stability with both heads locked together.

By using the wrist to move the ophthalmoscope, it is possible to examine the entire posterior retina without changing this basic position.

After examining the right eye, the examiner should switch the ophthalmoscope to the left hand and left eye to examine the patient's left eye from the patient's left side.

Some examiners may have such powerful ocular dominance in one eye that they will see the patients left ear with their right eye when trying to examine the left retina with their left eye. (Most people are right eye dominant. The opposite may apply if they are left eye dominant.) If this is the case, the examination with the ophthalmoscope can be delayed in the examination until the patient is lying on their back during the physical exam. With the patient lying down, staring at a dot or adhesive tape *X* on the ceiling, the right eye can be examined using the right eye, cheek to cheek.

> (Having the patient look at a ceiling light may constrict the pupil, making the visualization of the retina more difficult. Lowering the light level, by turning off lights in the room, will facilitate the examination of the retina.)

After examining the right eye, cheek to cheek, the examiner moves to the head of the exam table and examines the patient's left eye with the examiner's right eye from above the head, cheek to brow. The examiner must remember that the left eye appears upside down and backward. The left thumb may be used to lift the upper eyelid.

> My father, a general practitioner, lost his left eye as a teenager. He used this system to examine the retinas of every patient.

Examining the patient's left eye with the examiner's right eye in an upright position, nose to nose, is awkward. It is impossible to avoid bad breath and more likely that the examiner will catch any infectious disease that the patient may have.

> Another way to solve the ocular dominance problem is to use the wrist of the hand holding the upper eyelid to block the vision of the eye not looking through the ophthalmoscope.

The examination of the inner eye is much easier through a large pupil. Light from the ophthalmoscope will cause the pupil to constrict unless it is dilated pharmacologically.

There are many drugs that will dilate the pupil. They differ in rapidity of effect and duration of dilation. Some dilate the pupil without significant effect on accommodation. Most will block accommodation for hours to days.

The most commonly used dilating drop in most doctor's offices is Mydriacil (Tropicamide) 0.5%. One or two drops will dilate the pupil in fifteen to twenty minutes for a duration of three to six hours and block accommodation for thirty minutes to two hours. Neo-Synephrine (phenylephrine) 2.5% eye drops will dilate the pupil without blocking accommodation but must be used cautiously in patients with hypertension. The mydriasis (dilation) created will last up to six hours. Neo-Synephrine will cause blanching of the vessels of the conjunctiva, which should not be mistaken for systemic anemia.

Before using dilating drops, the anterior chamber depth should be determined to avoid causing a narrow angle glaucoma attack. See penlight examination.

A bottle of Mydriacil will be good for four weeks after it is opened, so it can be used on many patients if sterile technique is followed.

Examination of the Ocular Fundus

The term *ocular fundus* describes the posterior structures in the eye. These include the optic nerve head; the retina, including the nerve fiber layer; the retinal vessels; the choroid; and the vitreous adjacent to the retina. The area of the optic nerve and macula is referred to as the posterior pole of the eye.

To begin the examination, the nerve head (optic disk) is examined for color, shape, central cupping, position, and size of the vessels on the nerve head, and sharpness of the edges of the disk. The nerve should be slightly pink or yellow. Aspirin white and smooth denotes an atrophic or dead nerve.

The edge of the disk should be sharply demarcated. Fuzzy edges are caused by edema of the nerve in optic neuritis, as in multiple sclerosis or by elevated intracranial pressure causing papilledema, which appears out of focus and blurred.

The myelin sheaths of the nerve fibers in the optic nerve usually end at the cribriform plate of the sclera where the nerve enters the eye. In some patients, the myelin sheaths extend into the eye and spread from the optic disk, giving an irregular but distinct, edge, and a white appearance to the disk.

The nerve fibers curve into the optic nerve as they leave the eye, leaving a dimple in the center of the nerve. Glaucoma causes death of the nerve fibers of the optic nerve. This appears first in the middle of the disk with enlargement of the dimple into the optic cup. The vessels hug the edge of this cup and are displaced as the cup enlarges as more fibers are killed by the glaucoma. In advanced glaucoma, the chronic pressure causes the cup to extend posteriorly and to blow out of the eye and assume a bean pot shape. The holes in the cribriform plate may be visible at the bottom of the cup. The vessels arising in the center of the nerve may disappear behind the rim of the disk and reappear somewhat displaced from where they disappeared as they follow the walls of the cup. This is called bayoneting of the vessels.

Some patients will have a crescent of darker tissue or white sclera on one side of the disk where the retina and/or choroid is pulled away from the nerve head, allowing the choroid or sclera to show through. This is common in people with a high degree of myopia, so it is called a myopic crescent. In highly myopic people, it can occur all around the disk.

The retina is the only place in the body where vessels can be examined directly.

The ophthalmic artery and ophthalmic vein should emerge from the center of the disk and divide immediately into upper and lower branches. These immediately divide into temporal and nasal branches. In about 14% of eyes, there is a separate small artery that emerges from the temporal side of the disk to supply the retina between the disk and the macula.

Veins are larger than the arteries with a ratio of 4 or 5 to 3. In young patients, the examiner is actually seeing the column of blood within the vessels. The arteries are bright red, and the veins are dark red to purple. The vessel walls are transparent and only seen when they are abnormal.

When a vessel wall becomes atherosclerotic, it is opaque and partially blocks the view of whatever is beneath it. This is best seen where arteries cross over veins. The vein disappears in a gap between the arterial blood column and the venous blood column, because the vessel wall is blocking the view of the venous column. This is called gapping.

The arteries and veins on the retina share a muscular coat wherever they cross. In vascular hypertension, the increased tension in the artery wall squeezes the vein, pinching it as it passes under the artery. This appears as a notch out of the venous blood column or narrowing as it passes under the artery. This is called notching or nicking.

Veins usually cross the arteries obliquely. The pinching of the veins in hypertension causes them to cross perpendicular to the arteries. This is called banking of the veins.

Hypertension and atherosclerosis are often seen together causing a combination of these signs. Arteries with advanced atherosclerosis change color from bright red to a copper wire appearance. The bright line of light reflection from the top of the artery becomes brighter and wider. Arteries are narrowed in hypertensive patients, changing the ratio of vein diameter to artery diameter toward 2 to 1.

To maintain an orderly examination of the retina, the examiner should follow each of the four major branches from the disk to the periphery, noting the appearance of each crossing of artery and vein. The retina along the sides of each branch of artery and vein is examined for hemorrhages, exudates, abnormal pigmentation, and A-V crossing defects. The crossing defects are most visible when arteries cross over veins.

As the arteries bifurcate, the internal diameter decreases. Emboli from the carotid artery may enter the eye through the central retinal artery. Depending on the size of the embolus, they may lodge at the first arterial bifurcation, causing a central retinal artery occlusion or in a branch retinal artery causing a branch occlusion. The plaque causing the occlusion may be seen at the end of the blood column in the occluded artery. It appears as a white spot or light reflection.

The retina beyond the occlusion is usually pale because of lack of blood flow and the edema caused by anoxia. The anoxia of the vessel, caused by the blockage, may cause the artery distal to the blockage to dilate, which allows the plaque to move out further along the artery. Retinal artery occlusion is a medical emergency because the retina can only tolerate anoxia for ten to twenty minutes before the retina becomes permanently blind.

The appearance of the retina immediately after central retinal artery occlusion is striking. The retina becomes edematous and appears white. The fovea part of the retina is very thin, so the amount of edema that collects there is minimal and does not block the color of the choroid which appears red. The classic description of the retina in central artery occlusion is white with a cherry-red spot in the middle.

Occlusion of the central retinal vein is characterized by scattered hemorrhages throughout the posterior retina and dilated veins. The most common cause of central retina vein occlusion is arterial hypertension. Arterial hypertension also causes scattered flame shaped hemorrhages on the retina. Other causes of blockage to consider are blood hyperviscosity syndromes and diabetes.

The recording of the location and size of areas of hemorrhage or neovascularization is by direction from the disk and the number of disk diameters from the disk. The examiner looks at the disk and remembers the width of the disk and then estimates the number of disk diameters, edge to edge, that the lesion is located from the disk. The direction is by quadrant direction (e.g., superior temporal, inferior nasal, etc). For large hemorrhages, the size of the hemorrhage is compared to the size of the disk.

The earliest sign of diabetic changes in the eye is slight dilation and straightening of the veins. Diabetes also involves the small vessels within the retina. Capillaries dilate to become micro-aneurysms. The largest one-tenth of these can be seen with the ophthalmoscope as sharp-edged red dots. When damaged vessels break, they form round hemorrhages with fuzzy borders. These are called blot hemorrhages, like ink spots on a blotter or fabric.

Blockage of capillaries may cause small white fluffy infarcts of the retina called cotton-wool spots. When larger areas of the retina are compromised, the retina produces vascular endothelial growth factor (VEGF). VEGF causes new vessels to grow on the surface of the avascular retina and around the disk. These vessels are fragile and may lead to major hemorrhages within the vitreous. The hemorrhages organize into opaque sheets that are white or French's mustard yellow. Depending on the location of these sheets, they may block some or all vision.

Diabetic patients may have an unusual type of hemorrhage. This hemorrhage occurs between the retina and the posterior surface of the vitreous body. The hemorrhage dissects a circular space between the retina and the vitreous. When the patient sits or stands upright, the red blood cells settle to the bottom half of the space making a semicircle of red blood with clear fluid in the top half of the space. This is called a boat-shaped hemorrhage. The blood creates a blind spot that has the same shape as the hemorrhage, which is reversed, top to bottom, and left to right.

Retinal vessels branch repeatedly and are rarely straight, but tortuous snake-like vessels usually indicate pathology. This pathology (tumor or A-V malformation) may be beyond the part of the retina that is visible with a direct ophthalmoscope. Noticeable tortuosity should prompt a thorough exam by indirect ophthalmoscopy. (See later chapter.)

The retina away from the vessels should be examined for abnormal color, scars, and irregular pigmentation. The color of the retina is influenced by the skin color of the patient. Albino patients may have a very pink or red color. Blonds show a yellow color, while brunets show an orange background color. Black and brown patients may have a very dark orange to brown background color. Scars of the retina may be black or white with black edges and scattered pigment within the scar. Patients with high myopia or congenital toxoplasmosis may have large scars involving the whole central retina. Trauma to the eye may cause linear scars from tears in the choroid, which appear white because the retina lies directly on the sclera where the choroid is torn.

Scattered pigment in the mid-peripheral retina, which appears like bone spicules under a microscope, is seen in retinitis pigmentosum, a genetic disease of the retina that manifests during the teen years and progresses slowly, over the years, to total blindness.

After the other parts of the retina have been examined, attention is turned to the macula. By this time, the patient has usually become adapted to the bright light of the ophthalmoscope and should be more cooperative with the light on the fovea. The macula is aligned horizontally with the lower half of the disc and between two and three disk diameters temporal to the disk. It is the center of the circle formed by the superior and inferior temporal retinal arteries. It is easily recognized as the area where these arteries end in an avascular zone. There should be a cone shaped depression, the fovea, which is visible as a light reflection from the wall of the depression known as the foveal light reflex. Macular edema from trauma or diabetes causes this light reflection to disappear and may cause the fovea to be hazy or pale.

Older people are prone to retinal drusen. These are white spots in the pigment epithelium layer that are more common in the macular area. These white dots may be precursors of age-related macular degeneration (ARMD or AMD). The presence of drusen and scattered pigment with or without scars in the macula and with or without pallor of the retina (retinal edema) may be ARMD.

When examining the retina, the anatomy of the choroid and abnormalities may become apparent. The choroid is a vascular network that is very richly pigmented. The vascular network is fed posteriorly by several arteries that penetrate the sclera around the optic nerve and anteriorly by arteries that follow the extraocular muscles and penetrate the sclera near the muscle attachments. The choroid is drained by four vortex vessels that emerge in each quadrant between the muscles and slightly posterior to the equator of the eye. The vortex collecting veins may be visible as red lines in the darker background color of the retina.

The pigment in the choroid determines the color of the retina. Lack of pigment in an albino patient causes the white sclera to show through the retina making the fundus pink or white. Albino patients may have a poorly developed macula with no foveal light reflection. Blonds have light colored retinas while brunettes have a darker fundus. (This is independent of the color the hair on the head, if it is dyed.)

The pigment cells in the iris and choroid may give rise to pigmented nevi, which are characterized by being flat and uniform in brown or black color. These nevi must be followed because they may become a malignant melanoma. Melanomas may be thicker and vary internally in color. Testing with radioactive uptake can be used to differentiate a melanoma from a hemorrhage or nevus. When following a nevus, the size and location are very important. Many ophthalmoscopes have a light source that has a grid that projects in the light circle on the retina. This can be helpful in producing a sketch of the nevus shape. Optical changes in the eye, like cataract extraction, may change the size of the grid, so it is not reliable in determining growth. The location of nearby vessels should be recorded in the sketch so that changes in the relationship of the nevus to those vessels can determine growth.

Other alterations to the light source usually include a green light which is known as the red-free light source. Using the red-free light causes the vessels and hemorrhages to appear black, giving them more contrast with the retina to make them more visible. The red-free light is also considered a more monochromatic light. Monochromatic light may produce interference patterns in the nerve fiber layer. These are seen as tiny dark lines that run parallel to the nerve fibers. Loss of these lines may indicate loss of the nerve fiber layer from infarcts or glaucoma. This is esoteric and seldom used.

Another light source on some ophthalmoscopes is a straight line or slit beam. This is intended to act as a slit lamp beam. Looking straight down the light beam, as when examining the retina, defeats the purpose of the slit beam, which is best viewed at an angle to separate layers and accentuate differences in elevation. This light source can be used to examine the anterior chamber. When shown from the side, at a forty-five degree angle, the cornea appears as a curve. The beam should intersect the iris in a straight line. If the area of iris illumination is curved to the side, the anterior chamber is shallow and this pupil should not be dilated. If the iris is against the back of the cornea, the eye is probably in an angle closure glaucoma attack.

This ophthalmoscope slit beam can be used as an oblique light source to evaluate the lens of the eye (not looking through the aperture). It may reflect from the anterior or posterior surface of the normal lens. If the lens is hazy between the capsule surfaces, there is translucency of the lens. When this opacity is dense, there is a cataract forming in the lens. If the lens is white or brown, it is a cataract. The cataract will also interfere with the redness of the pupil when the full light of the ophthalmoscope in shown directly into the pupil and viewed through the aperture from several inches in front of the eye.

The routine physical examination of the eye is not complete without some estimate of the intraocular pressure. This is done by gently pressing on the eyeball through the upper eyelid with the eye is closed. The examiner should place both index fingers, side by side, on the upper eyelid, above the lid crease, and press gently on the eyeball, one finger at a time. The eye should be somewhat compressible. If it feels like a marble under the eyelid, the pressure is very high. The examiner can determine what feels normal by feeling many eyes, over time, including the examiner's own eye. Ophthalmologists learn to do this fairly accurately by comparing what they feel with the results of more accurate methods such as the Schiotz tonometer or the Goldmann applanation tonometer. These will be discussed in a later chapter.

Examination of Crossed Eyes (Strabismus).

Evaluation of ocular movements can be done at the beginning of the eye exam before examination of the retina or separately. Both active and passive movements should be evaluated.

The patient is asked to look right and left, up and down, up to the right and left and down to the right and left to evaluate active movement of the eyes. Passive movement is elicited by having the patient follow the light of a penlight to the same positions while the examiner watches the eyes. The eyes are observed to determine whether they are both looking at the object or if one eye deviates from looking at the object seen by the other eye. In small children, a toy, especially a noisy one, will attract and hold attention better. Failure to move into any of these positions deserves further examination to sort out the involved muscle.

Deviant eye movements may be caused by paralysis from nerve damage or from strabismus which is defined as intermittent or constant lack of parallelism of the visual axes of the eyes. Strabismus involves over- or under-action of one or more muscles.

Separating the ocular muscles involved in acute palsies was covered in the penlight exam.

Evaluating strabismus requires cover texting. Cover testing is done with both eyes open. The examiner directs the patient to look at a fixation target. (a letter on the eye chart, a light, a spot, or picture on the wall or any object directly in front of the patient, not to the side).

The examiner checks the ocular alignment to determine if both eyes appear to be looking at the object of regard. A cover (occluder, card, hand, etc.) is placed in front of one eye while the examiner watches the other eye. If the observed eye moves to look at the object of regard, it was not looking at the object before and was out of alignment. This is a tropia. The cover is removed and the eyes are watched. If the eye that is being uncovered moves, it had drifted behind the cover at the time when the uncovered eye moved to pick up fixation. (Both eyes moved together.)

There are several responses. If the eye being uncovered does not move, it may be suppressed and not seeing while the other eye is maintaining fixation. This is also a tropia. If the eye being uncovered moves and the eye that was not covered does not move, the patient is using both eyes and has fused the images from each into a single image. If the deviation is present only when one eye is covered, but recovers fusion when both eyes are open, it is a phoria.

Each eye is covered and uncovered to observe whether one eye is preferred after fusion is interrupted and then allowed to refuse.

If the eyes appear to remain straight during cover/uncover testing, the examiner proceeds to alternate cover testing. The patient looks at the object of regard while the examiner covers one eye and then the other so that one eye is always able to see the object of regard, but not allowing both eyes to see the object simultaneously. The examiner watches for movement in the eye being uncovered. If the eyes have a tendency to move away from parallelism when one is occluded but are held in place by neural muscular feedback from the brain that causes fusion of the two images when both are uncovered, the blocking of the image of one eye will allow that eye to move into its natural alignment. By alternating fixation by moving the occluder back and forth several times, the eyes will move to their preferred position. The deviation may increase in magnitude until the preferred position of the eyes is obtained. Deviation that is induced only by alternate cover testing and eliminated by allowing the eyes to fuse the two images is called a phoria.

Cover testing may cause a dissociated vertical deviation. This occurs when one eye is covered and the two eyes dissociate. The eye under the cover will move upward under the eyelid. When the eye is uncovered, it picks up fixation and returns to straight ahead. In some cases, the eye that is not covered will turn up away from the vision chart. To avoid this movement, the peripheral vision on the blocked eye must be maintained by covering the pupil with a thin cover such as a pencil or split tongue blade. This maintains peripheral fusion while blocking the chart and allows the eyes to stay in a forward looking position.

The name of the phoria or tropia is determined by the direction of the deviation. If the eyes move toward each other, it is called an *esophoria* or *esotropia*. If the eyes move away from each other, it is called an *exophoria* or *exotropia*. If the eye movement is vertical, it is called a hypertropia and named for the higher eye (i.e., right hypertropia when the higher pupil is in the right eye).

The term hypotropia is reserved for when the pathology is only in one eye, and it causes the eye to be pulled down, as in a blowout fracture of the orbit that has entrapped the inferior rectus muscle or ligaments, pulling the eye down, or from thyroid disease involving only one inferior rectus muscle that holds the eye down.

Hypertropias may be caused by oblique muscle over actions or under actions. These are brought out by passively moving the eyes to extreme lateral gaze and watching the pupils for vertical movement. The superior oblique muscle normally pulls the eye down, while the inferior oblique muscle normally pulls the eye up. The deviation is greatest in the field of action of the paretic muscle and least when the involved muscle should be relaxed.

Oblique muscle imbalance causes a rotational mal alignment of the images of the two eyes. The patient often develops a head turn or head tilt to put the involved muscle at rest, relaxing it similar to a paralysis therefore minimizing the deviation and diplopia. Sorting out these tilts and turns as well as recognizing Duane's retraction syndrome and Brown's superior oblique tendon sheath syndrome are left to more advanced texts.

Prisms may be used to determine the amount of deviation in strabismus. These are used in conjunction with cover testing. There are sets of single prisms of varying power or prisms assembled into prism bars. One bar has the prism power arranged vertically and another bar has them arranged horizontally when the bars are held vertically in front of the eye.

A prism approximating the amount of deviation is selected and held in front of one eye. Alternate cover testing with increasing or decreasing prism power is used to determine what prism power is needed to stop the movement of the eyes during alternate covering. Depending on the residual movement, the prism is increased or decreased until the prism neutralizes the movement of the eyes on alternate covering.

When both horizontal and vertical deviations are present, a prism is used in front of one eye to neutralize the vertical component.

A second prism is placed before the other eye to neutralize the horizontal component. This may require more than two hands to hold two prisms and move the cover, so an assistant may be needed. The measurement for strabismus is the prism diopter. (One prism diopter will deviate an image that is one meter from the prism by one centimeter toward the base of the prism.)

Children with accommodative esotropia have crossed eyes because they are very farsighted. They must accommodate (focus) to see clearly at distance. The synkinetic near response requires the eyes to turn inward when they focus. This makes them turn in when focused at distance and turn in more for near focus. They soon learn to turn off (suppress) one eye to overcome the diplopia. A suppressed eye may develop amblyopia (lazy eye). Removing the need to accommodate at distance will often allow the eyes to be straight at both distance and near. One tipoff to this diagnosis is the inability to get consistent measurements of the amount of strabismus. Once a prism correction is placed in trial frames on this patient, the strabismus remains variable. Under correction of the hyperopia does not straighten the eyes consistently, but full correction will usually work unless the esotropia is longstanding.

There are several instruments that can be used to measure the deviation of strabismus called troposcopes. These usually have one eye look at part of a picture (a clown) and the other eye look at the other part (balloons) through prisms or movable arms. The patient is instructed to align the images to make one picture (the clown holding the balloons). The angle of deviation is read from the instrument.

Rotational diplopia, caused by oblique muscle problems can be measured by placing Maddox rods in front of both eyes in a trial frame. With the patient looking at a point of light through the Maddox rods, the lenses are rotated by the patient until the streaks produced by the Maddox rods are aligned parallel. The angle of deviation can be determined by the relative position of the lenses.

# The Ophthalmic Slit Lamp

The slit lamp is an instrument that is designed to examine the eye in three dimensions with magnification. Because of the optical clarity of the cornea, lens, and intraocular media, the deeper parts of the eye can be examined through the more superficial parts using a thin slit bean of light.

The light source is a variable width beam of light that can be introduced into the eye at various angles to the axis of the eye and the viewing direction. In the anterior half of the eye, this slit beam produces an optical section of the eye. The image appears to be a thin slice through the eye like a section on a microscope slide. If the beam enters from the patient's right, the more anterior parts of the eye will be seen to the right in the section. The more posterior parts will be seen to the left.

The slit beam is used in conjunction with a binocular low power microscope for three dimensional viewing of the optical section under magnification. This magnification can be changed within the microscope by click-stop lens changes or a zoom lens, depending on the slit lamp, and also by changing the power of the oculars on the microscope.

When the eye is looking straight ahead with the beam coming in from the right, the anterior surface of the cornea will be at the extreme right of the section (light beam). The light passes through the cornea where some light is scattered, making the corneal stoma visible. As the light strikes Descemet's membrane and the corneal endothelium, it is reflected from these surfaces. As the beam passes through the anterior chamber, the aqueous humor is normally optically clear and does not reflect the light. When the beam intersects the iris, it illuminates the surface for examination through the binocular microscope.

If the beam is passed through the pupil it will reflect from the anterior capsule and pass through the visible cortex and nucleus of the lens to reflect from the posterior capsule. In the infant, the body of the lens is optically clear and may show very little light scatter, making it relatively invisible. By the teenage years, the lens cortex becomes more visible. By middle age, the nucleus becomes more visible than the cortex, which is also visible. As a cataract develops, the lens may become white or yellow, especially in the center or nucleus. Dense cataracts may be white or brown. Longstanding cataracts may appear black.

By definition, a *cataract* is opacity within the crystalline lens of the eye. Cataracts may develop anywhere within the lens. Scanning the slit beam horizontally may detect small dots, layers, streaks, or zones of opacity, or general haze.

A common type of cataract is called the posterior subcapsular cataract because it forms granules on the anterior surface of the posterior capsule (inside the lens). These granules increase in number centrally and spread from the center of the capsule toward the periphery.

Another type of cataract is the senile cataract. The nucleus and cortex of the lens become hazy.

Varying the width of the slit beam is useful in evaluating different parts of the optical section. A narrow beam is best for separating the various layers of the cornea to look at opacities within the cornea, such as the deposits of corneal dystrophies. A narrow beam allows accurate determination of the depth of scars, foreign bodies, and inclusions.

When evaluating corneal edema or the condition of the corneal endothelium, a wider beam shows the presence of pathology. Corneal edema is seen as whiteness of the band of epithelium illuminated by the beam. Tiny pockets of fluid within the epithelium, known as bullae, will appear as black dots in this cloudy band. The edges of cornea abrasions can be seen by light reflection within the beam. Subepithelial cysts or microscopic lines may only be seen with a wide beam.

Examination of the corneal endothelium requires a wide beam to see deposits or spots known as gutatta. These appear as a beaten metal surface or as dew on glass. A classic term for this is *bedewing* of the cornea. Inflammation within the eye may cause visible clumps of white blood cells to collect on the endothelial surface of the cornea.

Visualization of the surfaces of the lens is also best done with a wide beam to light up the surface. Position or depth of opacities or foreign bodies can be determined best with a narrow oblique beam that emphasizes depth by splaying the optical section horizontally.

The slit beam is usually mounted so that the beam passes through the optical center of the focal point of the microscope. Most slit lamps have the ability to move the beam away from this location. Moving the beam so that it shines on the limbus while the microscope is viewing the central cornea will bring out corneal edema, edges of epithelial defects, flaws in the stroma like tiny scars or empty blood vessels, and imbedded clear foreign bodies. This technique is known as scleral scatter.

Another way to facilitate examination of the cornea is by retro-illumination. The slit beam is directed to the front surface of the iris behind the area of the cornea to be viewed while the microscope is focused on the cornea. The light from behind brings out irregularities like pigment or cells on the endothelium, and gutatta, as well as corneal edema and corneal abrasions.

Most slit lamps have the ability to rotate the slit from the vertical position. This can be helpful to bring the slit across an ulcer or other lesion. It is also useful during gonioscopy, the use of a lens to examine the angle structures where the cornea, iris, and ciliary body come together. This area is important in glaucoma. The slit beam is rotated until it is perpendicular to the portion of the angle being viewed.

When the slit beam is rotated to the horizontal position, the microscope looks down the beam so there is no separation of the layers. Releasing the light source or moving the light source prism will allow the beam to tilt vertically, splaying the optical section to separate it in three dimensions for viewing. This is valuable for gonioscopy at three and nine o'clock and for examination of the vitreous.

Examining the Eye with a Slit Lamp

The slit lamp is a very useful tool for detailed examination of the eye and adnexa. The cost of a slit lamp makes it beyond cost effectiveness of most general physicians's offices, but slit lamps may be found in some emergency rooms. The slit lamps found in emergency rooms are used by most ER physicians to find and remove foreign bodies or examine ulcers on the surface of the cornea.

For ophthalmologists and non-ophthalmologists, the initial examination of the eye should be done in an organized, thorough, and disciplined manner. Skipping randomly from one part of the eye to another, in no particular order, is a recipe for missing pathology.

For a more detailed exam, progressing from the penlight exam to examination by slit lamp is logical next step. With the patient sitting in the examination chair, the slit lamp can be rolled or swung into position in front of the patient. Some offices have the slit lamp between stools for the patient and the examiner.

The patient is asked to lean forward to place their chin on the chinrest and their forehead against the forehead band. The height of the slit lamp can be adjusted up of down for the comfort of the patient. If the patient is uncomfortable, they will be less cooperative and the examination may be compromised. Most slit lamp tables have hand holds attached to the frame of the chinrest. Many patients are more comfortable holding these handles. To have the eye in focus, the patient must hold their forehead firmly against the forehead band. The chin rest can be adjusted so that the eye is aligned vertically with the slit beam. Most slit lamps have a line on the vertical part of the head rest to indicate the level of the slit beam, (level of the eye to be examined).

Buxom women may have trouble placing their chin on the chinrest. If possible, the slit lamp can be lowered or the patient elevated so that the patient leans forward to extend the chin forward ahead of their bosom. The head must tilted back from the axis of the spine to be upright in the slit lamp. This can be a problem in arthritic patients. Portable slit lamps are made for this situation.

The examiner can adjust the exam chair height and the height of the examiner's stool to be able to look through the binoculars of the slit lamp. The examiner places one hand on the joy stick that moves the slit lamp and uses the other hand to hold the head or eyelids of the patient, when necessary.

Children have a tendency to pull back from the slit lamp and may have to be gently held by the back of the head to keep their forehead against the forehead band. The patient is asked to look at the examiners ear with the eye that is not being examined. This will hold both eyes steady. The patient's gaze can be directed to the right and left as necessary to examine the sides of the eyeball.

While looking through the binoculars of the slit lamp, the examiner uses the joy stick to advance the slit lamp until it is in focus on the right eyelids. Looking through the microscope while moving the joy stick from side to side, the eyelid margins are examined, first the lower eyelid followed by the upper eyelid. The lashes are examined for regularity of spacing, length, direction, and color. The lid margin is examined for smoothness of the edge, notching, swelling, abnormal pigment, and presence of the grey line that runs along the middle of the edge. The openings of the meibomian glands should be visible, but not be inflamed, elevated, or plugged. The lacrimal puncta in each eyelid are identified and examined for patency. Gentle pressure with the examiner's index finger on the skin over the inferior-nasal orbit should not express mucus or pus from the punctum but may produce clear fluid. The eyelid should be congruent with the eyeball with a meniscus of tears spreading from the eyelid to the eyeball along the lower eyelid.

Using the hand on the same side as the eye being examined, the thumb is placed on the cheek to pull the lower eyelid down. The edge of the eyelid is examined for smoothness and aberrant lashes. Pulling the lower eyelid down further, the conjunctiva on the back of the eyelid can be exposed and examined for color, swelling, abnormal vessels, and depth of the cul-de-sac. Adhesions between the eyelid and the sclera may stand out as the lower eyelid is retracted.

The upper eyelid is examined for the same factors as the lower eyelid. Then examine the edge of the eyelid. The examiner uses the thumb of the hand on the side being examined to draw the loose skin of the eyelid up toward the orbital rim. This rotates the edge of the eyelid toward the examiner.

If there is a question of a foreign body behind the upper eyelid, the slit lamp is removed to access the patient to evert the eyelid. Holding the everted eyelid in place, using a thumb on the lashes against the brow while the patient is repositioned at the slit lamp, the conjunctiva on the tarsal plate is scanned using the joystick. Foreign bodies can be removed with a cotton-tipped applicator or small needle (insulin or TB syringe).

Attention is then directed to the conjunctiva. The caruncle should be smooth and pink. It may have spots on the surface. Next to the caruncle is the semi lunar fold which should be clear and grossly avascular with a sharp edge where it meets the conjunctiva of the eyeball. The patient is asked to look up to expose the lower conjunctiva. Having the patient look right and left will expose the nasal and temporal areas. Using the index finger or thumb to roll the upper eyelid upward against the superior orbital rim while the patient looks down, exposes the upper conjunctiva. A few small vessels are normal, but the conjunctiva should be clear and appear white because of the underlying sclera.

The nasal and temporal conjunctiva is examined for pterygia and pinguecula (described above) and abnormal pigmentation. The limbus, the junction of the cornea and sclera where the cornea curves forward from the spherical plane of the sclera, is the location where carcinoma of the conjunctiva is most often found. Hyperemia of the first two millimeters of conjunctiva from the limbus is called ciliary flush which is indicative of corneal disease or intraocular inflammation. Diffuse inflammation of the conjunctiva is usually indicative of bacterial or viral conjunctivitis or a glaucoma attack.

The slit beam is then directed to the cornea. The temporal cornea is best examined with the slit beam coming from the temporal side. The beam is then swung to the nasal side to examine the nasal cornea. The cornea is scanned for surface irregularities, scars, filled or empty blood vessels, pigment, and clarity, swinging the beam from side to side as needed. It is best to start with a sweep with the observer's scope set at low power for a general impression before switching to high power for detail.

Using a medium width beam, the epithelium is inspected for edema or blisters and the clarity of Descemet's membrane and the endothelium. The beam is narrowed to evaluate the thickness of the cornea and any abnormality of curvature such as keratoconus. Using a wider beam, the surface of the epithelium is evaluated for smoothness and clarity. Irregularities in the epithelium, such as abrasions or edema, will be obvious at this magnification and illumination. The stroma is inspected for inclusions from dystrophies, crystals from gout or dystrophies, scars from trauma or ulcers, or vessels from interstitial keratitis (TB or syphilis) or prior ulcers. The endothelium is examined for Descemet's tears or gutatta.

Gutatta are best seen by inspecting the area of brightest reflection of the slit beam. Gutatta will appear as dents in the smoothness of the reflection. They can also be viewed as distortion of the reflected light from the iris using retro-illumination while focused on the endothelium.

Before leaving the cornea, the knob holding the slit beam centered is loosened to allow the beam to be moved to shine on the limbus while examining the whole cornea. This illuminates the cornea from the inside, bringing out abnormal lines, (either anterior or posterior), edema haze of the epithelium, or reflective inclusions within the stroma. The slit beam is recentered and narrowed to use it to estimate the depth of any inclusions or vessels found.

Centering the slit beam and shining it through the edge of the cornea at three o'clock and nine o'clock, perpendicular to the cornea, allows the examiner to evaluate the depth of the anterior chamber. The ratio of the distance the slit travels through the peripheral cornea, compared to the distance from the inside of the cornea to the surface of the iris is noted. The distance from the cornea to the iris should be equal to or greater than the thickness of the cornea to consider the angle open normally. Care must be taken when using dilating drops for the pupil in an eye with a narrow angle and should be done only by an examiner capable of treating an angle closure glaucoma attack.

Aqueous humor in the anterior chamber is normally optically clear (dark). Inflammation causes a cellular and protein response in the aqueous humor. Cells appear as reflective specks floating in the fluid, like dust in the sunshine. Protein makes the aqueous hazy making the light path appear like headlights through fog. This is called flare. Cells and flare are graded by using a spot beam. Slit lamps have different ways to control the height and width of the beam. By narrowing both parameters, or using smaller apertures, a spot beam can be produced. The brightness of the haze (flare) and the number of cells within the bean are graded (1 to 4+) and recorded. Progress of the disease and/or therapy is determined by increases or decreases in the number of cells or the degree of flare.

If there is a layer of white blood cells in the lower anterior chamber it is called a hypopyon. The amount of white cells can be measured using the slit beam. The beam, in a vertical position, is placed over the hypopyon with the bottom of the beam at the limbus at six o'clock. The height of the beam is adjusted so that the bottom of the beam is at the limbus and the top is aligned with the top of the hypopyon. Changes in the height of the hypopyon, read on a scale on the slit lamp, indicate progress of the disease and treatment.

Hemorrhage into the anterior chamber, called a hyphema, will usually settle to form a layer in the lower anterior chamber, if the head is upright. It can be measured in the same way as the hypopyon. The absorption or recurrence of the hemorrhage can be followed by this measurement of the height of the hyphema. If part of the blood is clotted, the height of the settled portion is still relevant. If the patient lies on their back, the blood will settle on the iris and the amount of blood cannot be determined. The height of the blood will be most accurate if the patient has been sitting upright for fifteen to twenty minutes for the blood to settle.

Attention is directed to the surface of the iris. The joystick is used to sweep the beam across the iris, observing the anatomy and texture of the iris surface. It should be lacy and uniform in color. In a dark-colored iris, pigment may cover the iris and fill the holes in the lacy stroma making it appear smooth. The central iris is thinner than the periphery. The edge of the thicker part is usually demarcated by a circular drop off called the collaret. A pigment ring may be obvious at the edge of the pupil where the posterior pigment layer may be seen. After inflammation in the eye, the iris may become adherent to the lens, either at local spots or for up to 360° around the pupil. These adhesions may prevent the pupil from dilating when the slit beam is narrowed to decrease the light stimulus to the eye. This response to light can also be tested by moving the slit beam alternatively through the pupil and away from the pupil onto the iris.

Pigmented spots may occur on the surface of the iris. These may be solitary or multiple. They are more obvious on light colored irises, but appear as smooth, solid spots on the lacy background of the iris stroma. These should be noted and diagramed in the record, so that growth can be detected. In an eye clinic, photographs of nevi are taken to be placed in the record for future comparison. Color change or growth should suggest the presence of a melanoma or metastatic cancer.

White or gray flakes may appear on the surface and crypts of the iris stroma and at the edge of the pupil. A deposit that appears like peeling paint may be seen on the surface of the lens. This layer is missing in a circle on the surface that corresponds to the range of movement of the pupil edge as it dilates and constricts under normal lighting conditions. The edges of the peeling material are cracked and elevated. The flakes have been described as dandruff of the iris. This is called a pseudoexfoliation cataract. These flakes may drift into the trabecular meshwork, blocking it and creating a glaucoma situation.

Holes, other than the pupil, may occur in the iris. These may be congenital or from a diseases process. The name for this is polycoria. The actual pupil will constrict normally to light stimulus, but abnormal holes will sometimes show a paradoxical response as they are pulled open as the true pupil constricts.

The iris contains both radial and circular muscles for dilation and constriction of the pupil, but they are not usually visible. They may be seen in an atrophic iris (i.e., after anterior segment necrosis).

The blood supply consists of radial and circumferential vessels, which are imbedded in the iris stroma and therefore not visible. On rare occasion, in the presence of extraordinary inflammation, the vessels dilate and appear as red spirals or corkscrews within the lacy stroma.

When the slit beam is directed obliquely through the pupil, the front surface of the lens is illuminated. It will appear as a curved stripe in the slit beam. Light passing through the lens will be scattered by the cortex and nucleus of the lens as a hazy media. Brighter lines or zones may be seen in the slit beam; these represent the interface of the cortex and nucleus or signs of maternal disease during development of the lens *in utero*. Two *Y*-shaped stars may be seen within the lens, representing the lines where cortical fibers meet at the center of the lens as they arch around the nucleus from front to back. The bodies of these cells are centered on the equator of the lens with the tips of the cells extending anterior and posterior in the lens. One of these *Y*s is upright, the other upside down.

Small white spots may occur randomly in the body of the lens. These are technically congenital cataracts that do not usually interfere with vision. Maternal illness during gestation, such as measles or syphilis, may cause layers or zones of the cells to be partially or completely opaque, forming what is called a zonular cataract.

At the back of the lens, the slit beam illuminates the posterior capsule as a band of reflection. Posterior sub-capsular cataracts begin as granules on the posterior capsule at the center of the capsule. These may be seen as dots against the red reflection created by reflected light from the retina. Direct examination with the slit beam shows them as white or pearly spots anterior to the capsule. These spots may become confluent as a growing solid spot on the capsule.

Senile cataract formation causes the nucleus to become white or yellow. The yellow turns to brown and, if allowed to remain in the eye, it may become black. Maturation of the cataract causes the cortex to turn white and liquefy, allowing the nucleus to sink to the bottom of the lens. Using a very narrow beam, the nucleus can be seen in the bottom of the capsule within the milky liquefied cortex. This is described as the "setting sun" sign of a hyper mature cataract.

When the lens is relatively clear, the anterior vitreous can be seen behind the lens. Fibers may be seen swishing around within the eye as the eye moves. Having the patient look right and left or up and down will accentuate this movement of the vitreous. Dense membranes from old, organized, intraocular hemorrhage from trauma or diabetes may appear as white or French's mustard yellow sheets. These usually block the red reflection from the retina and block the view of anything behind the membrane. These membranes are usually avascular. A membrane with vessels is usually a detached retina that has pulled forward within the eye.

The slit lamp can be used to examine the clarity and position of surgically placed intraocular lenses and the lens capsule after intra-capsular cataract surgery. It is also used for minor surgical procedures, such as removal of superficial foreign bodies, or a needle-knife opening of clouded lens capsules after cataract surgery, called a capsulotomy. The slit lamp can be used for the delivery of laser beams for capsulotomies, glaucoma treatments, or laser applications to the retina for diabetic retinopathy or retinal detachment.

Slit Lamp for Examination of the Posterior Eye.

To see further into the eye, past the lens, it is necessary to use special lenses to overcome the light bending of the cornea. Some slit lamps come with a Hruby lens mounted on the slit lamp. This is a very high minus lens that neutralizes the positive power of the cornea and lens. To examine the retina with a Hruby lens, it is necessary to dilate the pupil as widely as possible. The Hruby lens has the disadvantage of making the image small.

The slit beam is directed through the Hruby lens at the pupil with a slight angle to one side or the other. To look at the optic nerve, it is best to introduce it from the temporal side since the nerve head is nasal to the macula. This beam will light up vitreous strands or sheets and will give the examiner a profile of the surface of the retina and optic nerve. The beam may be used to illuminate the cup of the disk to determine the depth and shape of the cup in the nerve. Using minimal light and a very narrow beam, the posterior surface of the vitreous can be seen if it has separated from the surface of the retina. Vitreous is slightly more translucent than the fluid that collects between the vitreous and the retina after posterior vitreous detachment. This separation occurs normally during the seventh or eighth decade of life in humans. Examination of the macula may reveal a hole in the macula caused by vitreous traction when posterior vitreous detachment is incomplete, leaving a vitreous attachment to the macula.

Large contact lenses with angled mirrors mounted within the lens are used to examine the macula, the posterior perimacular area, mid-periphery, and anterior periphery of the retina using different mirrors. The macula and optic nerve are examined through the center of the contact lens. The slit beam and viewing are directed in to the mirrors to illuminate and examine the peripheral retina. The contact lens is rotated to examine the entire retina. The slit is kept perpendicular to the mirror so that the slit remains within the area viewed through the mirror. To accomplish this, the slit is rotated using the rotation system of the slit lamp. When looking at three o'clock and nine o'clock, it is necessary to tilt the beam above horizontal so that the light section made by the beam can be viewed from an angle.

Another approach to viewing the retina with a slit lamp uses as high plus lens that is held in front of the eye. These lenses range from sixty to ninety diopters in power or higher, giving different amounts of magnification. The plus lens creates a virtual image that is viewed by the examiner through the slit lamp optics. The advantage of the high plus lens is higher magnification of the retina with greater ease of detecting pathology. Some examiners find it harder to use the high plus lenses than the contact or Hruby lenses.

The slit lamp is also used to view the angle structures where the iris and ciliary body meet the sclera. This technique uses a contact lens containing a mirror that is angled to look immediately behind the cornea. Some gonioscopic lenses use three mirrors to examine the angle, the peripheral retina and the equatorial retina.

When the slit beam is directed through the cornea toward the angle without the contact lens, the light is reflected by the anterior and posterior surface on the cornea and cannot reach the angle. The contact lens is placed on the cornea using a viscous solution to fill the space between the lens and the cornea to negate the reflective optical surface of the cornea.

To place this large contact lens in the eye, the concave surface of the lens that will be against the cornea is filled with a viscous solution. The eye is anesthetized with drops. While the examiner holds the lens in one hand, the patient is instructed to look up. The lower eyelid is retracted with the thumb of the examiner's other hand. The edge of the lens is held against the eye just above the lower eyelid and then quickly rotated upward to place the concave surface against the cornea. The patient is told to look straight ahead while the lens is held firmly against the eyeball. This will center the lens over the cornea. On some lenses, a flange on the lens will hold the eyelids to help hold the lens against the eye.

By shining the beam onto the mirror positioned on the opposite side of the eye from the angle being viewed, the light can pass through the cornea and illuminate the angle structures and reflect back out through the negated corneal surface. The optical property of the lens also makes it possible for the angle to be viewed through the mirror. The lens is rotated on the eye, lubricated by the viscous solution so that all parts of the angle can be seen. By having the beam at a slight angle, the structures are separated for observation.

If the angle is open, there is space between the iris and the cornea, the trabecular meshwork, Schlemm's canal, the sclera spur, and the anterior surface of the ciliary body and iris can be seen. Attachments of the iris to the cornea or trabecular meshwork, called anterior synechiae, can be seen. Trauma to the eye may cause the aqueous to dissect through the trabecular meshwork or between the sclera and choroid, leaving a tear or cleft. This may lead to traumatic glaucoma that occurs from weeks to years after the trauma. This cleft can be seen by using gonioscopy.

Some patients have blood vessels that cross the angle from sclera to iris in the far periphery. These are usually not significant, but they can cause hemorrhage in the eye if an anterior chamber lens is placed in the angle where one of these vessels occurs.

If the angle is closed, the iris is against the back of the cornea, so the angle structures cannot be seen. Angle closure occurs rapidly in angle closure glaucoma, but slow and chronically after prolonged uveitis that causes anterior synechiae that attach the iris to the cornea. Angle closure glaucoma with high intraocular pressure usually causes corneal edema that blocks the view of the angle. Hypertonic topical glycerin solution applied to the cornea before placing the gonioscopic lens will usually clear the cornea sufficiently to allow gonioscopy.

As a cataract matures, it may swell and push the iris forward toward the cornea narrowing the angle and creating a situation in which the angle can close when the pupil dilates in dim illumination.

Testing for Glaucoma.

The early stages of chronic simple glaucoma are symptom-free The pressure is low enough that it does not cause pain and the visual defects do not appear until there is significant damage to the retina. Screening for elevated intraocular pressure is very important. Experienced examiners can palpate the eyeball through the eyelids and determine if the pressure is within the normal range. Using a calibrated instrument is much more accurate.

The instrument that is most readily available to the general physician is the Schiotz tonometer. This is a handheld instrument with a central cylinder that ends in a curved faceplate. The cylinder contains a central plunger that protrudes from the faceplate. The other end of the plunger rides against a movable needle that moves along a calibrated arc. The needle points to numbers on a curved scale indicating the amount of indentation of the cornea produced by the plunger when the instrument is rested upon the eye. This scale reading is converted to pressure within the eye using a table supplied with the tonometer. This is similar to testing a bicycle tire by in indenting it with a thumb.

To use the Schiotz tonometer, the patient must be lying supine, facing up or in a reclining chair with the head facing up. Because the tonometer will touch the eye, it is necessary to anesthetize the eye with topical 0.5% proparacaine eye drops, or similar. The patient is asked to look at a fixation target (a spot on the ceiling or their own thumb held at arm's length, directly above their eye). The examiner retracts the eyelids of the eye to be tested using the thumb and middle finger against the cheek and eyebrow, being careful not to put pressure on the eyeball.

The tonometer is held vertically with the other hand using the small handles that hold a slide on the cylinder. The tonometer is brought in front of the eye, from the side, being careful not to obstruct the vision of the other eye that is looking at the fixation target. By bring the tonometer from the side, it is out of focus and not as much of a threat to the patient. If the tonometer is brought down toward the eye from above, the patient will reflexively try to close the eye to protect it.

The tonometer is centered over the cornea and gently lowered until it rests on the eye and its weight is not supported by the hand of the examiner. The position of the needle on the arcuate scale is read. If the reading is below the second mark of the arc, more weight is added to the plunger and the measurement is repeated. The process is repeated for the other eye, exchanging the hands holding the eyelids and the tonometer. The tonometer should be sterilized before use with alcohol or ether, being careful that no solution is left in the space between the plunger and the outer cylinder. This sterilizing solution will damage the cornea with a painful burn if allowed to contact the cornea.

Most ophthalmologists use an applanation tonometer that is attached to the slit lamp called a Goldman applanation tonometer. This instrument has a truncated cone with a flat front surface that is used to flatten the surface of the cornea. The force necessary to flatten a given area of the cornea is proportional to the amount of pressure within the eye. The dial on the tonometer is calibrated in millimeters of mercury pressure (mmHg) within the eye.

The cone is mounted so that turning a knob on the base unit applies increasing pressure on the eye. The cone contains a prism that splits the image of the flattened circle horizontally into two half circles. By aligning the split circles so that the opposite edges of the circles align (left edge to right edge), the flattened area has reached the predetermined amount. The pressure is read from the knob on the base unit. The edge of the circle is difficult to see, so fluorescein is placed in the tear film along with topical anesthetic. The tear film containing the fluorescein is squeezed from between the cone and the cornea and forms a ring around the flattened area, accentuating the edge of the flattened area. The green semicircles are aligned so that they just touch at the internal edge.

After the placement of the fluorescein and topical anesthesia, the patient is placed at the slit lamp. The patient is instructed to look at the examiner's ear with the eye not being tested. The light on the slit lamp is set to blue to make the fluorescein glow green. The applanation cone is brought toward the center of the cornea until it touches the cornea and the green ring is seen. The knob on the base unit of the applanator is turned until the edges of the split circle are aligned. The applanator is retracted from the eye and the pressure is read from the knob. This is repeated with the other eye. The tip of the cone is immediately wiped with alcohol or other sterilizing solution to avoid transmission of infections. (The number one reason for pink eye from adenovirus is recent tonometry.)

This same principle is used with the air puff tonometer. A jet of air is blown at the cornea to flatten the central cornea. A light is shown at an angle at the cornea. The airstream is delivered with increasing force. The duration of the pulse determines the flattening of the cornea. When the cornea has been sufficiently flattened, the light will reflect off the cornea toward a sensor. The time until the light is reflected the correct amount to hit a sensor on the opposite side of the eye is calibrated to the pressure applied. That pressure is displayed by the instrument.

The air puff tonometer does not require topical anesthetic, so it is preferred by optometrists. Patients who are familiar with the test are often wary of the air puff and tend to anticipate it by drawing back from the instrument just as the puff occurs, causing inaccurate results. Some patients refuse the test because it startles them.

There is an electronic applanation tonometer that uses a strain gage or change in inductance to determine the pressure applied when the correct area has been flattened. This tonometer can be used anywhere on the cornea or sclera. This system has been adapted to the handheld Tonopen that is slightly larger than a fountain pen. Handheld applanation tonometers have also been developed that use the prism and Fluorescein method of the Goldmann applanator in a portable unit.

# Visual Fields

The visual system of the eye is not limited to straight ahead. Each eye can usually see sixty to seventy degrees to the nasal side of straight ahead and nearly ninety degrees to the temporal side (150° total). The vertical visual field extends about 50° up and 70° down from horizontal. The refraction of light by the cornea allows vision to the far periphery when not obstructed by the nose, cheek or brow. The central areas of the two eyes, up to 60° in all directions from straight ahead, overlap and constitute the area of three-dimensional vision. Since the fields of the two eyes overlap, blind spots up to a hemiretinal area (nasal or temporal) in one eye may be overlooked by the patient. It is necessary to evaluate each eye individually to check for partial loss of the visual field of each eye. Bitemporal hemianopia from pituitary disease affecting the optic chiasm (damaging the crossing nasal retina nerves, leaving only the nasal half fields in both eyes) may not be noticed by the patient since the field is relatively full when both eyes are open.

To test major field loss, the patient is seated in front of the examiner with one eye covered. This cover can be an eye patch, the palm of the patient's hand held over the eye, or a facial tissue drawn behind the glasses to block the vision in one eye. The patient is instructed to look at the examiner's nose and not to peek to the side. The examiner reaches both hands beyond the patient's head and asks the patient to tell when they see a finger coming into the periphery of their visual field. One hand is brought forward toward the center until the patient reports seeing it. The hand is moved up and down around the circle of the visual field to text multiple meridians. This is called confrontation field testing. The examiner notes where the hand comes in further than usual.

If there is suspicion of major visual field loss, that is not found by simple confrontation. The examiner presents two hands in front of the patient simultaneously in two different quadrants and asks the patient to count the total number of fingers held. The examiner holds up one, two, or four fingers on each hand (three fingers are confusing) and asks the patient how many fingers they see all together. Mistakes in the number of fingers seen will pick up subtle field loss after vascular occlusions or strokes, or extensive field loss from glaucoma. This is called simultaneous two quadrant confrontation field testing.

Dr. J. Lawton Smith, a famous neuro-ophthalmologist, used an umbrella with a white laser pointer to check visual fields of bed ridden patients. He held the open umbrella above the patient and moved the light image of the laser pointer around the inside of the umbrella to determine the extent of the visual field.

More formal visual fields that are used for therapeutic decisions can be done with a tangent screen. This is a large flat panel that is covered with black felt that is on a stand or mounted on the wall. There is a white spot or button in the center of this screen for visual fixation.

The patient, with one eye occluded, is seated before the screen with a distance of one meter from their eye to the fixation point at the center of the screen. The patient is told to keep looking at the central white spot while the examiner uses a black wand to introduce graduated sized white spots from the periphery toward the center of the screen. The patient is instructed to tell the examiner as soon as they see the spot. Using the largest spots first allows the patient to learn the procedure and prepares them for smaller spots.

Black pins are placed in the felt to record the point where the spot was seen or the locations are recorded on a standard field chart. This is done from all directions until a perimeter of the field is mapped. The spot is changed to a smaller spot and the process repeated for several spot sizes. These perimeters are recorded on a standard visual field chart. Most ophthalmologists use colored pencils to record the different spot sizes.

There are various visual field testing devices that use an arc of the spherical field to present the spots from the periphery toward the center of vision. The arc can be rotated to plot the various meridians of the visual field.

This was replaced with a perimeter device called a Goldmann perimeter that has a large spherical bowl with a light projector to present white spots on the inside of the bowl. The examiner sits behind the bowl and watches the patient's eye through a telescope to be sure that the patient does not look for the spot. The pointer device is moved on a visual field map that is mounted behind the bowl in order to bring the light spot from the periphery toward the center. The field map is marked with dots when the patient reports seeing the spot. These dots are connected to show the perimeter for that spot size. Various spot sizes are mapped to determine visual field status.

These bowl perimeters have been automated using computers to present spots randomly and monitor the position of the patient's eye. The spots can be varied in size and brightness to map thresholds of visual perception throughout the field.

For very sensitive testing of central visual field loss from situations like Plaquenil toxicity causing visual loss when treating lupus, rheumatoid arthritis, dermatomyositis, and long-term malaria prophylaxis, visual field testing, using red targets is very useful. This will reveal very subtle visual loss before loss is detected by the usual visual acuity testing. More modern means of screening include OCT (ocular coherence tomography) and multifocal electroretinography.

Many states require a horizontal visual field of at least 100° with both eyes open to get a driver's license. This is tested with a one centimeter white spot. At the license office, this is often tested using a one meter arc mounted above the examining chair that has a one centimeter white ball, hung by a black rod from the end of the rotating rod. The examinee is seated beneath the rotating rod. The spot is introduced from the far right and rotated forward until it is seen. The number of degrees from straight ahead is recorded. The ball is then introduced from the left and rotated forward until it is seen. The number of degrees from straight ahead is noted and added to the first measurement to determine the total horizontal field, with both eyes open.

This number can be determined from formal visual fields by adding the furthest right vision in the either eye to the furthest left vision in either eye.

Measuring Ocular Proptosis or Exophthalmous

When the patient has prominent, bulging eyes it is important to quantitate the extent of the protrusion of the eye anterior to the lateral orbital rim to be able to judge progression or regression of the disease. The instrument used to measure this is called an exophthalmometer. There are two designs of equipment for making this measurement.

One is a clear square rod that is calibrated in millimeters from the pointed end. It is called a Luedde ophthalmometer. The rod is held perpendicular to the facial plane with the pointed end pressed against the lateral orbital rim. Sighting through or over the clear rod, the profile of the eye is seen. The position of the front surface of the cornea is read from the calibrations on the rod. Care must be taken to look through or over the rod parallel to the facial plane to avoid errors of parallax. This system is available with two rods mounted on a cross bar. The two rods are pressed against both lateral orbital rims. The protrusion is read from each side, being careful to avoid parallax.

This system can be approximated with a small millimeter ruler. The end of the ruler is held against the outer orbital rim and the protrusion measured by sighting across the face from the side.

The other system uses two 45° prism mirrors that are mounted on a crossbar so that the profiles of the eyes can be seen through the prisms. The tips of the mounting bracket are placed against the lateral orbital rims. The profile of the eye is viewed from in front of the patient through the prisms. Red lines on the prism must be aligned to avoid viewing from an angle that creates parallax. When the two red lines are superimposed, parallax error is eliminated. Each eye is read separately. The examiner is positioned in front of the patient throughout this procedure and can observe that the patient is looking straight ahead during the measurement. To assure that the ophthalmometer is placed in the same way for repeat measurements, there is a scale on the telescoping lockable crossbar to assure that the frame rests at the same position when this measurement is repeated. The amount of protrusion for each eye and the setting of the crossbar are recorded for each measurement.

# Central Retinal Arterial and Venous Pressure

The ocular fundus is the only place in the body where blood vessels can be viewed directly without opening a body cavity. The ophthalmic artery is the first artery that branches from the internal carotid artery. The venous pressure in the central retinal vein is influenced by intracranial pressure and pressure in the superior vena cava. The effects of hypertension, arteriosclerosis, diabetes, carotid emboli and intracranial pressure can be seen directly in the vascular system of the eye.

One of the signs of elevated intracranial pressure is absence of the spontaneous pulsation of the central retinal vein. Elevation of the intraocular pressure caused by glaucoma may accentuate spontaneous pulsation of the central retinal vein. Pulsation of the central retinal vein in a normal eye can be produced by finger pressure on the eyeball—directly on the sclera or through the eyelids. This pressure can be quantitated using an instrument called an ophthalmodynamometer. This instrument has a spring loaded plunger that is connected to a movable slide or circular dial to record the pressure in the eye. Using a direct ophthalmoscope, or the indirect ophthalmoscope, the observer watches the central retinal vein where it emerges from the center of the optic nerve while applying pressure to the sclera with the tip of the plunger of the ophthalmodynamometer. (Topical anesthesia is required.) The examiner applies increasing pressure against the eyeball until the vein starts to pulsate and then immediately reduces the pressure. The slide or dial marks the maximum of the pressure applied. The reading from the instrument is converted to mmHg by a table, supplied with the instrument, to determine venous diastolic pressure. The ophthalmodynamometer is reapplied to the eye, increasing the pressure until the vein collapses completely and stays closed, indicating that systolic venous pressure has been reached. This reading is converted on the table to determine venous systolic pressure in mmHg.

> (Using a contact lens to observe the vessels on the
> optic nerve may introduce pressure or vacuum to the
> surface of the eye, so it is not recommended.)

The same procedure can be used to determine the diastolic and systolic pressure in the central retinal artery. It is not recommended to occlude the central retinal artery completely for more than a few seconds to avoid damage to the retina or occlusion of the vessel. Near total obstruction of the internal carotid artery or ophthalmic artery by atheromatous plaques may significantly reduce central retinal artery pressure. Comparison of the central retinal arterial pressure in the two eyes may indicate partial carotid stenosis that is greater on one side.

The Indirect Ophthalmoscope

The indirect ophthalmoscope is an ingenious way of looking at the retina by viewing a virtual image of the retina that is formed in front of the eye. Because the image is a virtual image, it is upside down and reversed right to left.

A high plus lens is used to condense the light reflected from the retina into the virtual image. This allows a three dimensional vision and a wide field of view of the retina and ocular contents. The image is viewed through special lenses and prisms in the headset that decrease the interpupilary viewing distance of the headset so that both eyes can see through the dilated pupil.

If enough light can be reflected from the retina, even through a cataract, the virtual image may be sufficient to "see" the retina through the cataract. The optics of the lens allows the examiner to see almost the entire retina by having the patient look in all of the cardinal directions. By gently pressing on the sclera to indent the anterior retina with a sclera depressor or a Q-tip, the anterior edges of the retina and part of the ciliary body can be seen. (It is difficult to see the equator or further anterior parts of the eye with the direct ophthalmoscope.) The indirect ophthalmoscope allows the examiner to find the anterior holes in the retina that cause retinal detachments and pathology in the anterior retina. The wide field of the indirect ophthalmoscope is at the cost of magnification which is nil. The examiner must constantly remember that the image is upside down and backward. (The invention of the indirect ophthalmoscope revolutionized repair of retinal detachments, because all of the anterior holes causing the detachment could be visualized and closed.)

When using the indirect ophthalmoscope, the patient may be sitting or lying in the supine position, staring at the ceiling. The pupil must be dilated unless a special "small pupil" scope is used. The examiner places the headset on the head and adjusts the light and adjusts the interpupillary distance prisms to fuse the images and light beam straight ahead.

The examiner directs the light beam into the pupil to obtain a red reflection from the retina. The lens in then held in the light beam and moved around until the image of the retina is seen, filling the lens ring. The lens is moved closer to, or farther from, the eye until the image is in focus. The patient is directed to look right, left, up, and down or places in between to bring the peripheral retina into view. The examiner moves around the patient to see various parts of the retina. The retina is examined for abnormal pigment, coloration, vascular patterns, and holes. Holes appear as red spots under the absent retina and may be round, linear, or horseshoe shaped. Scars from prior disease or laser treatment may be white or black, depending on the pigment distribution.

The examination can be done with the patient seated, but this position limits the movement of the examiner with respect to the view of the eye.

This sounds fairly straight forward, but it is difficult to align the light beam, the lens, and the pupil to create an image without significant amounts of practice. Neophytes may see the retina by looking through the observation mirror/prism while an experienced ophthalmologist examines the retina.

The indirect ophthalmoscope can be used to visualize the retina when there is partial opacification of the cornea, lens, or vitreous body such that the retina cannot be seen with a direct ophthalmoscope.

# Poor Man's Indirect Ophthalmoscope.

If the pupil is dilated, as it is after surgery, the retina may be viewed using an indirect ophthalmoscope lens and a penlight. The penlight is held against the examiner's temple or just below the line of vision and directed at the pupil. The handheld lens is held in front of the eye and positioned to create the virtual image. This method works to check the macula and optic nerve, but is difficult to use to see the peripheral retina. It is difficult to see the retina with both eyes simultaneously using this system, so the view is two dimensional. Detached retina is grey or white and can be differentiated using the poor man's ophthalmoscope if it is in the posterior eye.

# Index

fuzzy edges, 59

## G

gapping, 60
glands of Moll, 26
glaucoma, 59, 66, 77, 91, 96, 101
glycosaminoglycans, 42
Goldmann applanation tonometer, 67
Goldmann perimeter, 97
gonioscopic lenses, 89
gutatta, 76–77, 82

## H

hazy oil, 35
head tilt, 6, 27, 71
head turn, 71
hemorrhage, recording of the location
    and size, 62
hemorrhages, ix, 19, 39, 61–62, 66,
    83, 90
      boat-shaped, 63
heterochromia, of the iris, 23
high cholesterol, 22, 35, 43
high plus lens, 88–89, 102
hordeolum, 35–36
horizontal rectus muscles, 14
Horner's syndrome, 23
Hruby lens, 87, 89
Hudson-Stahli line, 45
hyper mature cataract, 86
hyperopia, 8, 44, 72
hypertension, 15, 61
hypertensive patients, ix, 61
hyperthyroid disease, 15
hypertropia, 70

hypervitaminosis A, 20. *See also*
    vitamin A excess
hyphema, 83
hypopyon, 46, 83
hypothyroid disease, 34
hypotropia, 70

## I

idoxuridine (IDU), 48
illiterate person, 9
indirect ophthalmoscope, 25, 52, 101–5
intraocular inflammation, 45, 81
intraocular pressure, 67, 90–91, 101
iris., 19

## J

jaundice, 20, 37
Jones II test, 49
Jones I test, 49

## K

Kayser-Fleischer ring, 22, 45
keratoconus, 44–45, 81

## L

lacrimal canaliculus, 28, 48
lacrimal duct, 49
lacrimal punctum, 28, 49
lacrimal sac, 28, 48–50
Lacrimal System, 46–48
lagophthalmos, 29
levator muscles, 27, 31
light reflection on the cornea, 11, 42
light response
    direct pupillary, 16

# U

upper eyelid, double eversion of, 32
upper eyelid fold, 27
uveitis, 23, 25, 46

# V

vascular endothelial growth factor (VEGF), 63
vascular hypertension, 39, 60
veins, ix–x, 60–61, 63, 65, 101–2
venous diastolic pressure, 101
visual acuity, 1, 4, 9
visual acuity test, 1–5, 7–9, 98
visual fields, 95–98
visual field testing, 97–98

vitamin A deficiency, 21
vitamin A excess, 37
vitreous, 24, 58, 88
Von Recklinghausen's disease, 34
vortex vessels, 65

# W

Weill-Marchesani syndrome, 25
Wilson disease, 22

# X

xanthelasma, 35

# Y

yellow sclera, 20
Y-shaped stars, 85